Transdiagnostic
LGBTQ-Affirmative
Cognitive-Behavioral Therapy

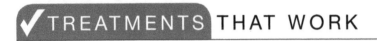✔ TREATMENTS THAT WORK

Transdiagnostic LGBTQ-Affirmative Cognitive-Behavioral Therapy

CLIENT WORKBOOK

JOHN E. PACHANKIS
SKYLER D. JACKSON
AUDREY R. HARKNESS
STEVEN A. SAFREN

OXFORD
UNIVERSITY PRESS

OXFORD
UNIVERSITY PRESS

Oxford University Press is a department of the University of Oxford. It furthers the University's objective of excellence in research, scholarship, and education by publishing worldwide. Oxford is a registered trade mark of Oxford University Press in the UK and certain other countries.

Published in the United States of America by Oxford University Press
198 Madison Avenue, New York, NY 10016, United States of America.

© Oxford University Press 2022

Library of Congress Cataloging-in-Publication Data
Names: Pachankis, John E. author. | Jackson, Skyler D., author. | Harkness, Audrey R., author. |
Safren, Steven A., author.
Title: Transdiagnostic LGBTQ-affirmative cognitive-behavioral therapy : client workbook /
John E. Pachankis, Skyler D. Jackson, Audrey R. Harkness, Steven A. Safren.
Description: New York, NY : Oxford University Press, [2022] |
Series: Treatments that work | Includes bibliographical references and index.
Identifiers: LCCN 2022018796 (print) | LCCN 2022018797 (ebook) |
ISBN 9780197643341 (paperback) | ISBN 9780197643365 (epub) | ISBN 9780197643372
Subjects: LCSH: Sexual minorities—Mental health. | Cognitive therapy.
Classification: LCC RC451.4.G39 P33 2022 (print) |
LCC RC451.4.G39 (ebook) | DDC 616.89/14250866—dc23/eng/20220510
LC record available at https://lccn.loc.gov/2022018796
LC ebook record available at https://lccn.loc.gov/2022018797

DOI: 10.1093/med-psych/9780197643341.001.0001

9 8 7 6 5 4 3 2 1

Printed by Marquis, Canada

One of the most difficult problems confronting people with various disorders and diseases is finding the best help available. Everyone is aware of friends or family who have sought treatment from a seemingly reputable practitioner, only to find out later from another doctor that the original diagnosis was wrong or the treatments recommended were inappropriate or perhaps even harmful. Most people, or their family members, address this problem by reading everything they can about their symptoms, seeking out information on the internet or aggressively "asking around" to tap knowledge from friends and acquaintances. Governments and health care policymakers are also aware that people in need do not always get the best treatments—something they refer to as *variability in health care practices*.

Now health care systems around the world are attempting to correct this variability by introducing *evidence-based practice*. This simply means that it is in everyone's interest that people get the most up-to-date and effective care for a particular problem. Health care policymakers have also recognized that it is very useful to give consumers of health care as much information as possible, so that they can make intelligent decisions in a collaborative effort to improve physical health and mental health. This series, Treatments *ThatWork*, is designed to accomplish just that. Only the latest and most effective interventions for particular problems are described, in user-friendly language. To be included in this series, each treatment program must pass the highest standards of evidence available, as determined by a scientific advisory board. Thus, when individuals suffering from these problems or their family members seek out an expert clinician who is familiar with these interventions and decides that they are appropriate, patients will have confidence they are receiving the best care available. Of course, only your health care professional can decide on the right mix of treatments for you.

LGBTQ people seek mental health care more frequently than the general population, likely because of the distinct stressors that they must navigate across their lives. Stressors such as coming out; forming an LGBTQ identity in a heteronormative, cisnormative world; the emotional legacy of early negative experiences; and internalized stigma show clear associations with several mental health conditions, including depression and anxiety. LGBTQ-affirmative cognitive-behavioral therapy is an evidence-based program specifically designed by and for LGBTQ people to address the impact that LGBTQ-related stressors can have on mental health.

LGBTQ-affirmative cognitive-behavioral therapy is designed to reduce symptoms of depression and anxiety, general distress, and co-occurring behaviors, such as high-risk substance use and sexual behaviors. This program teaches cognitive-behavioral skills that help people address the difficult emotions and avoidance tendencies underlying a spectrum of mental health concerns. Explanations are provided in each chapter for why certain techniques or practices can be specifically helpful for LGBTQ people as they work to undo the mental health challenges of LGBTQ-related stress and general life stress. LGBTQ-affirmative cognitive-behavioral therapy will be an indispensable resource for LGBTQ people interested in using cognitive-behavioral therapy to improve their emotional well-being, and in finding ways not only to navigate stressful challenges, but also to embrace the many gifts associated with being LGBTQ.

David H. Barlow, Editor-in-Chief
Treatments *That Work*
Boston, MA

Contents

Acknowledgments

The material contained in the therapist guide and client workbook for *Transdiagnostic LGBTQ-Affirmative Cognitive-Behavioral Therapy* derives from several sources. Most significantly, the *Unified Protocol for the Transdiagnostic Treatment of Emotional Disorders—Therapist Guide* and the *Unified Protocol for the Transdiagnostic Treatment of Emotional Disorders—Patient Workbook* by David Barlow, PhD, Todd Farchione, PhD, and colleagues served as the basis for the materials contained herein. David Barlow, PhD, Todd Farchione, PhD, and Oxford University Press provided permission to work from the Unified Protocol to prepare the *Transdiagnostic LGBTQ-Affirmative Cognitive-Behavioral Therapy—Therapist Guide* and *Transdiagnostic LGBTQ-Affirmative Cognitive-Behavioral Therapy—Client Workbook*. The general outline and much of the text about the nature of emotional disorders, setting goals, increasing cognitive flexibility, emotion exposures, and relapse prevention comes directly from the *Unified Protocol* Therapist Guide and Patient Workbook. John Pachankis, PhD, thoroughly revised and updated the outline and text of the *Unified Protocol* Therapist Guide to specifically respond to the needs of LGBTQ clients, including through consultation with LGBTQ community members and expert mental health providers, following an adaptation process described elsewhere[1]. This adaptation process resulted in the inclusion of LGBTQ-specific content throughout the therapist guide. Much of this new content focuses on the relevance of LGBTQ-related stress triggers and maladaptive coping responses as sources of emotional disorders for LGBTQ individuals. Other new content for *Transdiagnostic LGBTQ-Affirmative Cognitive-Behavioral Therapy* includes the chapter regarding functional analysis, which was influenced by[2] *Cognitive-behavior therapy: Reflections on the evolution of a therapeutic orientation*, and the chapter regarding experimenting with new

---

[1] Pachankis, J. E. (2014). Uncovering clinical principles and techniques to address minority stress, mental health, and related health risks among gay and bisexual men. *Clinical Psychology*, 21(4), 313–330.

[2] Goldfried's (2003).

reactions and assertiveness, which was influenced[3] *Responsible Assertive Behavior: Cognitive/Behavioral Procedures for Trainers*. The LGBTQ-specific adaptation of that specific approach is described elsewhere[4]. Mark Hatzenbuehler, PhD, contributed helpful suggestions at the adaptation stage.

The client workbook was created from several sources, starting with the therapist guide described above and session summaries of Transdiagnostic LGBTQ-Affirmative Cognitive-Behavioral Therapy created by Charles Burton, PhD, Melvin Hampton, PhD, Craig Rodriguez-Seijas, PhD, Ingrid Solano, PhD, and Katie Wang, PhD. Several individuals initially helped revise the therapist guide and these session summaries to use more easily accessible, client-centered language, based on their practical experience delivering the therapy in clinical trials. These individuals worked closely with John Pachankis, PhD, to undertake this initial language revision. The team included the following individuals: Charles Burton, PhD (treatment introduction, Chapter 2; goal setting, Chapter 4); Nitzan Cohen, PhD (introduction to LGBTQ-related stress, Chapter 5; relapse prevention, Chapter 12); Zachary Rawlings, PhD (understanding emotions, Chapter 6; emotional behaviors, Chapter 9; emotion exposures, Chapter 11); Kriti Behari, MA (awareness of LGBTQ-related stress reactions, Chapter 7); Tenille Taggart, MA (cognitive flexibility, Chapter 8; countering emotional behaviors, Chapter 11); and Alexander Belser, PhD (experimenting with new reactions to LGBTQ-related stress, Chapter 10). John Pachankis, PhD, subsequently edited these language revisions. Following this client-centered language revision process, Cal Brisbin, BA, Benjamin Fetzner, BA, Eric Layland, PhD, Erin McConocha, MPH, and Ilana Seager van Dyk, PhD, performed additional revisions to further increase language accessibility and LGBTQ relevance. These materials were then thoroughly edited and revised by John Pachankis, PhD, Skyler Jackson, PhD, Audrey Harkness, PhD, and Steven Safren, PhD,

---

[3] Lange, A., & Jakubowski, P. (1976). *Responsible assertive behavior: cognitive/behavioral procedures for trainers*. Champaign, IL: Research Press.

[4] Pachankis, J. E. (2009). The use of cognitive-behavioral therapy to promote authenticity. *Pragmatic Case Studies in Psychotherapy, 5*(4), 28–38.

taking into account subsequently published clinical trials results of this treatment[5–7], the revisions included in the second edition of the *Unified Protocol*, and alignment with the content of the therapist guide for *Transdiagnostic LGBTQ-Affirmative Cognitive-Behavioral Therapy*. Benjamin Eisenstadt proofread the therapist guide and client workbook and contributed style and content edits to both texts.

[5] Jackson, S. D., Wagner, L., Yepes, M., Harvey, T., Higginbottom, J., & Pachankis, J. E. (2021). A pilot test of a treatment to address intersectional stigma, mental health, and HIV risk among gay and bisexual men of color. *Psychotherapy*

[6] Pachankis, J. E., Harkness, A., Maciejewski, K.R., Behari, K., Clark, K. A., McConocha, E., Winston, R., Adeyinka, O., Reynolds, J., Bränström, R., Esserman, D. A., Hatzenbuehler, M. L., & Safren, S. A. (in press). LGBQ-affirmative cognitive-behavioral therapy for young gay and bisexual men's mental and sexual health: A three-arm randomized controlled trial. *Journal of Consulting and Clinical Psychology.*

[7] Pachankis, J. E., McConocha, E. M., Wang, K., Behari, K., Fetzner, B. K., Brisbin, C. D., Scheer, J. R., & Lehavot, K. (2020). A transdiagnostic minority stress intervention for sexual minority women's depression, anxiety, and unhealthy alcohol use: a randomized controlled trial. *Journal of Consulting and Clinical Psychology, 88,* 613–630.

CHAPTER 1 ▸ About This Treatment

Chapter 1 Overview

In this chapter, you will learn about LGBTQ-affirmative cognitive-behavioral therapy: where it came from, how it was developed, and how it can help to address some of the specific stressors you may face as an LGBTQ person. This chapter will introduce you to the concept of LGBTQ-related stress and the role that it can play in the emotional experiences of LGBTQ people.

Chapter 1 Outline

- What Is LGBTQ-Affirmative Cognitive-Behavioral Therapy and How Can It Help You?
- Why Have a Specific Therapy for LGBTQ People?
- The Principles of LGBTQ-Affirmative CBT
- How Should You Use This Program?
- What Are the Benefits of This Program?
- What Are the Potential Drawbacks of This Program?
- Summary

What Is LGBTQ-Affirmative Cognitive-Behavioral Therapy and How Can It Help You?

LGBTQ-affirmative cognitive-behavioral therapy, or CBT, is a mental health treatment created *for* LGBTQ people *by* LGBTQ people. It is based on the evidence-based techniques of CBT, a type of therapy that has a lot of research supporting its effectiveness.

This treatment is designed to help LGBTQ people who are experiencing emotional reactions or stressors in their lives. Emotional reactions or stressors can lead to worse problems such as depression, generalized anxiety, problematic substance use, or other persistent problems stemming from strong emotions such as obsessive-compulsive disorder or sexual behavior that feels out of control.

CBT is based on learning skills to manage distress. Each chapter in this workbook will introduce you to new CBT skills for managing your emotional experiences that might be directly or indirectly caused or worsened by stress related to being LGBTQ. This treatment program is designed so that each chapter builds upon the one before it, so you can practice each skill, see if it helps, and then learn the next new skill in the next chapter.

The treatment begins by reviewing the types of emotions that you might be currently experiencing. This treatment recognizes that some or much of your emotional experience might be directly or indirectly impacted by LGBTQ-related stress. You will learn:

- How to be more aware of your emotions and the stressors that cause them;
- How stressors impact your thoughts, feelings, and behaviors; and
- Specific ways to transform less helpful coping strategies into more helpful ones.

Although this treatment program focuses on stress related to being LGBTQ, you probably experience many different types of stress in your life. Some stressors, like work or school stress, may not be related to being LGBTQ or your identity. Other stress might be related to other parts of your identity, such as your race/ethnicity, religion, employment status, language, ability, or many other identities that can sometimes serve as sources of identity-related stress (and pride). This therapy can also help you with these other types of stress.

Why Have a Specific Therapy for LGBTQ People?

Research shows that LGBTQ people are more likely than heterosexual, cisgender people to experience mood and anxiety disorders because of the added stress LGTBQ people face. We call this stress "LGBTQ-related stress," although it is sometimes also called "minority stress."

Many LGBTQ people experience LGBTQ-related stress in their daily lives in obvious ways, like constantly fearing rejection because some family, friends, or members of society have rejected them in the past. LGBTQ people can also experience stress in less obvious ways, like not having the same social support as heterosexual or cisgender people. LGBTQ people might also start to believe negative ideas about themselves that they hear. For example, they might think that they are weak, unhealthy, or less important than heterosexual/cisgender people. They might even think about hiding who they really are because they are ashamed or afraid of how others might react. These processes can be quite subtle but ultimately accumulate over time to cause strong, uncomfortable emotional reactions. When stressful situations and interactions related to being LGBTQ happen over and over, many LGBTQ people start to feel like they have no control over the problems they face in their day-to-day lives. Feeling out of control and uncertain on a daily basis can lead to strong, uncomfortable emotional reactions.

This treatment program does not assume that all LGBTQ people have experienced all these types of stress. However, the program does recognize that the stressors that LGBTQ people face can lead to feelings of depression, anxiety, problematic drug use, and other emotional disorders.

This treatment will ask you to think carefully about the ways that LGBTQ-related stress might be contributing to your difficult emotional experiences. It will provide you with the tools you need to start changing the way you cope with this stress, and all stressors in your life, so that you can start responding to your emotions differently.

The Principles of LGBTQ-Affirmative CBT

LGBTQ-affirmative CBT has six core principles. You may already be aware of some, and others may be surprising. Take a moment to read them; they will be important throughout the treatment:

1. **Uncomfortable emotional experiences like depression and anxiety are normal responses to LGBTQ-related stressors.** How do you think this principle might apply to you? Maybe you've been

feeling depressed and anxious for a while and have been wondering what's wrong with you. We know that LGBTQ-related stress can be bad for mental health, and that it's OK to not be OK.

2. **Early and ongoing experiences with LGBTQ-related stress can teach LGBTQ people powerful and negative, yet faulty, lessons about themselves.** If you grew up or live in a culture that does not support LGBTQ people, you probably started to believe these negative messages in some way or another, maybe without even realizing it. You might believe (perhaps deep down) that you don't matter as much as heterosexual/cisgender people, that you don't deserve love, or that you are a bad person. These messages can become so deeply fixed that they can affect us in ways we don't even realize.

3. **LGBTQ people can effectively cope with the unfair results of LGBTQ-related stress.** You may not have control over the LGBTQ-related stress in your day-to-day life, but you *do* have control over how you cope with this stress. LGBTQ-affirmative CBT is designed to give you the information, tools, and support to try new ways of coping with LGBTQ-related stress.

4. **LGBTQ people have unique strengths.** Resilience and growth are often forged in the fires of adversity. The fact that you are reading this and trying out LGBTQ-affirmative CBT means that *you* have overcome major challenges in your life. Exploring your sexuality and/or gender identity is something that most people never have to do. The fact that you are willing to do that shows you are brave. Also, did you know that members of the LGBTQ community have been some of the most important thinkers, artists, and athletes in history? This treatment program is just one of many resources to help you use your strengths and achieve your goals in life.

5. **Sex is healthy!** You might have learned from a young age that sex is wrong, especially if you're sexually attracted to someone who identifies as the same gender as you. Shame around sex can lead to all sorts of problems, like using drugs to avoid feeling shame, having sex in a way that feels out of your control, or avoiding conversations about sex that probably would be helpful. Sex is a normal and enjoyable natural drive, and this program is designed to help you have the relationships, sexual or otherwise, that are most in line with your values and goals.

6. **Genuine, real relationships are essential for LGBTQ people's mental health.** LGBTQ-related stress might have made you feel lonely or unvalued in your early relationships. It may also be shaping your current relationships (even ones that are supportive of you

being LGBTQ!). For example, you might find it difficult to totally open up or "be yourself" around even your close friends because early on, LGBTQ-related stress made it seem like there are parts of you that should not be seen by others. This treatment program will help you figure out how LGBTQ-related stress may be making your relationships less than healthy. It will also give you the tools to change your relationships, and even make new ones. This is one of the most important things you can do for your mental health.

How Should You Use This Program?

If you are working with a therapist who is using this treatment program, you will likely meet with your therapist on a weekly basis, spending one or more hour-long sessions focusing on the content of each chapter in this workbook. Working with a therapist on this treatment program can be ideal, but this option isn't always available for everyone. Therefore, you might also be using this workbook on your own. If that is the case, then you can go through the workbook at your own pace. We recommend spending enough time on each chapter to really get comfortable using the skills. Each chapter also has exercises to help you practice the skills in response to strong emotions in your own life.

Note that practice is important! The practice activities for each chapter will help you use these skills in your real life. Practicing hard things can be a drag. But whether this treatment works really depends on how much effort you put into it. Think of it as deciding to enter a marathon. You can't just sign up and expect to be able to run the entire marathon without breaking a sweat. You have to start several months before, exercising a bit more every day, until eventually you build the muscles and the stamina needed to carry you through. Remember: Learning comes by doing! The more you practice the skills, the easier the skills will become.

What Are the Benefits of This Program?

This treatment is based on CBT a type of that has a particular focus on helping people better understand and respond to their emotional experiences. This CBT was developed at the Center for Anxiety and Related Disorders at Boston University and is rooted in many decades of research into the causes of emotional disorders and their effective treatment. Researchers have found that this type of CBT leads to significant improvements in the majority of people who undergo this therapy, and it helps them use the skills they have learned to better cope with their emotions. Additionally, many people who have received the treatment also report significantly improved ability to achieve goals in many aspects of their lives (e.g., improved relationships, improved performance at work).

Given the success of this type of CBT for the general population, clinical researchers at Yale University, working with the Yale Initiative for LGBTQ Mental Health, adapted this type of CBT to specifically address the concerns and emotional experiences of LGBTQ people. The Yale researchers enhanced CBT for LGBTQ people by consulting with dozens of clinical experts and diverse LGBTQ community members, as well as collaborating with other researchers who study LGBTQ mental health. Through this deep consultation process, they were able to create a CBT that specifically addresses LGBTQ-specific stressors and reactions. Across several clinical trials and several hundred LGBTQ people, this new LGBTQ-affirmative CBT is associated with reductions in depression, anxiety, substance use, and other emotional disorders.

Of course, we cannot promise that this treatment will lead to significant improvements for everyone. However, the biggest predictor of success is the amount of effort you dedicate to this program. The more you put into this treatment, the more you will get out of it.

What Are the Potential Drawbacks of This Program?

Like most important goals, changing how you cope with your emotions takes work. The biggest drawback of using this program is that to get something out of it, you need to put something into it: time and effort. You should be prepared to set aside time each day to practice the skills you're learning. Additionally, it is best if you continue to move through the skills without long breaks. Think of it like signing up for a course in school—for the three to four months you're enrolled, you are learning new concepts and regularly doing homework to practice what you have learned. If you are unable to make this commitment, it may not be the right time to try this program. In order to really give this program a chance to work, you should be willing to see it through from beginning to end. Keep in mind that many people feel nervous about committing to confronting difficult emotions. However, when they take it step by step, they often surprise themselves by how much they learn.

Summary

In this chapter, you learned about the rationale for LGBTQ-affirmative CBT: where it came from, how it was developed, and how it can help to address some of the specific stressors you may face as an LGBTQ person. This treatment program is designed for LGBTQ people who are currently experiencing uncomfortable emotions that over time can cause depression, anxiety, and related emotions and behaviors that cause distress. This chapter introduced the concept of LGBTQ-related stress and the role that it can often play in the emotional experiences of LGBTQ people.

The next chapter will introduce you to the relationship between LGBTQ-related stress and emotional disorders. The chapter will review how emotional disorders come about and the role that LGBTQ-related stress often plays. Chapter 2 will also introduce a systematic approach to understanding the reasons for different types of uncomfortable emotional experiences and the role that stressors play in maintaining these emotions. This approach will set the stage for you to treat your emotions differently through the helpful CBT skills contained in the remainder of this workbook.

Emotional Difficulties and
LGBTQ-Related Stress

Chapter 2 Overview

In this chapter, you'll learn about difficult, distressing emotions and
how negative reactions to strong emotions can actually make them
worse. You'll be introduced to new ways to respond to your emotions
that can ultimately help you feel better. This chapter also reviews the
ways that LGBTQ-related stress can contribute to distressing emotions.
The chapter ends by introducing you to the components of LGBTQ-
affirmative cognitive-behavioral therapy (CBT) that will be the focus of
this treatment.

Chapter 2 Outline

- When Do Emotions Get Too Distressing?
- How Does LGBTQ-Related Stress Contribute to Distressing
  Emotions?
- The STAIRCaSE Model of LGBTQ-Related Stress and Emotional
  Disorders
- Preview of LGBTQ-Affirmative CBT
- Home Practice: STAIRCaSE: Identifying When You Have Strong
  Emotions
- Summary

This treatment program was developed to help LGBTQ people who are struggling with distressing emotions. These emotions can include things like anxiety, sadness, anger, and even shame. Negative emotions can require treatment when they become overwhelming or they get in the way of moving forward in life. For example, feeling really sad may make it harder to reach out to friends or even get out of bed. Feeling anxious at school or work may prevent someone from finishing important tasks. You may have picked up this workbook because your emotions are interfering in your own life in ways that matter to you. Although emotions affect our lives in different ways, there are three features that often occur across all emotional disorders:

1. **Frequent, strong emotions:** People who struggle with emotional difficulties tend to feel strong emotions quite often. Research shows that exposure to chronic stressors, such as LGBTQ-related stress, can increase people's tendency to feel strong emotions. Some people also have a biological tendency for strong emotions—some people may simply be "hard-wired" to experience their emotions more intensely in response to situations in their lives. It is important to point out, though, that feeling emotions strongly does not necessarily mean a person will find them overwhelming and interfering. It is how we respond to our emotions that really matters.

2. **Negative reactions to emotions:** Sometimes people with emotions that are too distressing also tend to view having these emotions negatively. They can be hard on themselves for having certain reactions, thinking, "I shouldn't be feeling this way" or "Getting upset about this is a sign of weakness." They may also link strong emotions to bad outcomes and conclude things like, "Everyone will judge me for being anxious," "If I get angry, I'll do something that I'll regret," or "If I let myself feel sad, I'll fall into a hole that I won't be able to get out of." Sometimes one part of an emotional experience is particularly distressing. For example, some people may find the physical sensations associated with emotions, such as a racing heart, sweating, and butterflies in the stomach, quite uncomfortable. For others, intrusive, unwanted thoughts may be most difficult. Sometimes, people even have negative reactions to positive emotions (e.g., "If I let myself feel excited, I'll be even more disappointed if it doesn't work out").

As we discuss below, LGBTQ-related stress can also contribute to LGBTQ people's negative reactions to their emotions.

3. **Avoidance of emotions:** It makes sense that people with distressing emotions who view their emotions negatively would want to try to avoid having strong emotions. This is called "avoidance." The problem with avoidance is that it actually doesn't work very well and often even backfires. Actively trying to push away emotions may sometimes make you feel better in the short term, but generally leads to more frequent, intense emotions in the long term. It is like being stuck in quicksand—the more you struggle, the more you sink. Additionally, by avoiding activities or situations because they might bring up intense emotions, life can become limited. You may find it difficult to get the most out of day-to-day activities like going to work, spending time with friends, or just having fun.

Acceptance of Emotions: A Better Way

The goal of this workbook is to change the way you respond to your emotions when they occur. Specifically, you will be asked to approach your emotions in a more accepting manner instead of viewing them as something to avoid. This may seem like the opposite of what you are expecting because perhaps you are hoping to *get rid of* your overwhelming emotions. However, as you progress though this workbook, you will learn more about how emotions, even negative ones, are important, and that pushing them away actually hurts more than it helps. Leaning in toward your emotions and responding more effectively to them may be difficult at first, but it will gradually make them easier to deal with.

Over time, strong emotions can get in the way of a person's ability to live the life they want. Their negative reactions to their emotions are driving them to do things they don't want to do—and, as we'll discuss throughout this program, things that might make them feel better for a short time (e.g., skipping gatherings with classmates, snapping at a partner, rigidly following a routine) only lead to more problems in the long term. Over time, these strong emotions and people's ways of coping with them can create emotional disorders.

Emotional disorders occur when the way a person responds to strong emotions is taking over their life. Examples of emotional disorders include anxiety disorders such as panic disorder, generalized anxiety disorder

(GAD), social anxiety disorder (SAD), and obsessive-compulsive disorder (OCD). Depression is another common emotional disorder.

These disorders all share a common feature—a person's negative reactions to strong emotions. But by targeting negative, avoidant reactions to emotions, this treatment program can help you address all of the symptoms you are experiencing, regardless of the disorder.

Even if you have not received one of these formal diagnoses, this program might still be a good fit for you. If your emotions (or the strategies you use to manage them) are interfering with living the life you want to lead, you will probably benefit from the skills taught in this workbook. For some people, strong emotions affect nearly every aspect of their lives, while for others, difficulties with emotions only occur in one or two contexts (e.g., public speaking, romantic relationships). In fact, we think that everyone can benefit from learning healthy ways to respond to emotions! Either way, learning to be more accepting of emotions when they come up can help them become more manageable over time.

How Does LGBTQ-Related Stress Contribute to Distressing Emotions?

LGBTQ-related stress can contribute to emotional disorders in several ways:

1. LGBTQ-related stress adds to the general life stress that all people experience to increase the total level of stress that LGBTQ people experience. Because LGBTQ people experience LGBTQ-related stress in addition to everyday stress, such as stress related to work, school, relationships, and finances, they are more likely to feel the strong emotions associated with stress. Over time, this elevated stress and these strong emotions can give rise to emotional disorders.

2. LGBTQ-related stress can teach LGBTQ people that their emotions are bad, shameful, and something to be avoided. As noted above, one feature of emotional disorders is a tendency to have these negative reactions to one's emotions. These negative reactions can then actually worsen the emotions being experienced. LGBTQ people are often taught from an early age that the way they express themselves, including their emotions, is bad, wrong, and shameful. The message can be: "You should not feel the way you feel or act the way you act." Early and ongoing exposure to messages like this can make LGBTQ

people feel that they should not have the feelings they have or should not trust these feelings, listen to them, or express them. This type of invalidation of emotions can increase LGBTQ people's risk for emotional disorders.

3. Early and ongoing experiences of LGBTQ-related stress, especially experiences of rejection from family or peers or violence, can teach LGBTQ people that danger or threat of rejection is always lurking. Over time, LGBTQ people can start expecting danger or rejection even in seemingly safe situations, such as their own friendships or romantic relationships. As we will discuss below, chronically being on the lookout for danger or always expecting rejection can lead to emotional disorders.

The STAIRCaSE Model of LGBTQ-Related Stress and Emotional Disorders

At this point you might be thinking about the kinds of LGBTQ-related stress you have faced and may continue to face in your life. You might have also started making connections between that stress and the most pressing concerns that brought you to this treatment. This program uses an acronym called "STAIRCaSE" to help understand the connections between LGBTQ-related stress and emotional disorders (see Box 2.1 for an introduction to this model).[1,2] It can be helpful to think through, on your own and/or with a therapist, how this model applies to you. This section will guide you through each component of the model, with some questions to help you think through each step.

Figure 2.1 illustrates the STAIRCaSE Model of LGTBQ-related stress and emotional experiences.

Let's think through how each of the components of the model apply to your life. Use Worksheet 2.1: The STAIRCaSE Model at the end of this chapter to keep track of your answers to each set of questions. You may

---

1 Goldfried, M. R. (1995). Toward a common language for case formulation. *Journal of Psychotherapy Integration*, 5(3), 221–244. https://doi.org/10.1037/h0101272

2 Eubanks, C. F., & Goldfried, M. R. (2019). A principle-based approach to psychotherapy integration. In J. C. Norcross & M. R. Goldfried (Eds.), *Handbook of psychotherapy integration* (3rd ed., pp. 88–104). Oxford University Press. https://doi.org/10.1093/med-psych/9780190690465.003.0004

Box 2.1. What Does STAIRCaSE Mean?

The STAIRCaSE Model can help you think through how LGBTQ-related stress has affected your experience of strong, uncomfortable emotions. STAIRCaSE stands for:

S: The **Situations** that lead you to think unhelpful thoughts, experience strong emotions, or engage in behaviors that may be unhelpful (like avoidance). For many LGBTQ people, these situations include experiences with LGBTQ-related stress or situations that bring up memories of past LGBTQ-related stress.

T: The **Thoughts** that you have in these situations, including thoughts you have about your emotions. For many LGBTQ people, LGBTQ-related stress has an impact on the content and patterns of thoughts in these situations.

A: **Affect** is another word for emotions and here refers to the emotions/emotional experience you have in these stressful situations. These emotions might include fear, anxiety, sadness, anger, guilt, shame, and embarrassment. Affect also includes the physical component of uncomfortable emotions (e.g., fatigue, sleep problems, upset stomach).

I: **Intention** refers to what you need or want in these situations. For example, you might want to be able to express yourself authentically (i.e., "be yourself"), to be heard and respected by the other people in the situation, or to behave in a way that is consistent with your values. You also might want to not feel strong uncomfortable emotions. Intentions can also refer to your long-term goals or values (e.g., wanting to get in a relationship).

R: Your **Response** refers to what you do in situations to cope with whatever strong emotions arise. It is common for people with depression and anxiety to respond to these situations by avoiding, escaping from, or trying to control the uncomfortable emotions that the situation brings up. This kind of response can become a habit—meaning that every time a situation that triggers LGBTQ-related stress occurs, you are more likely to engage in the same behavior.

C: **Consequences** are what happens because of your response to the situation. There are usually both short-term and long-term consequences. When you respond to a stressor by avoiding it, the short-term consequence is that you have reduced your discomfort or stress. But, in the long term, avoidance can lead to negative consequences, such as keeping you away from your intention and leading you to view yourself in a more negative way.

SE: **Self-Evaluation** refers to how you see yourself and your performance in these challenging situations. Your self-evaluation also includes how well you feel you are able to cope with challenging situations, including those that cause LGBTQ-related stress.

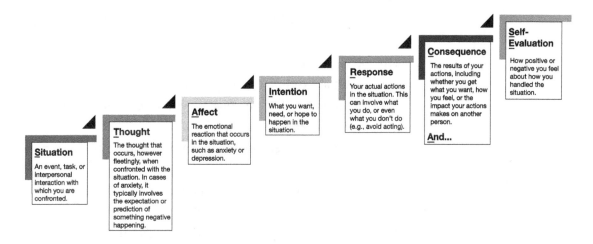

Figure 2.1

The STAIRCaSE Model of LGBTQ-Related Stress and Emotional Experiences
Figure created by Nicole Barle, Stony Brook University.

also download a copy of the worksheet by searching for this book's title on the Oxford Academic platform at academic.oup.com.

1. What **Situations** elicit LGBTQ-related stress for you?
   - What situations cause you to feel strong, uncomfortable emotions today? Who is there? What is taking place in these situations? When and where do they happen?
   - What has your experience of LGBTQ-related stress been in the past (e.g., when you were growing up)?
   - What about broader, more indirect experiences of LGBTQ-related stress you may have experienced—things happening at a societal level or in your community that may not have directly affected you, but still may have been stressful?
   - Have these situations occurred on multiple occasions? It is common for LGBTQ-related stressors to "add up" over time, making you feel worse.
2. What **Thoughts** are you experiencing in situations that trigger LGBTQ-related stress?
   - Do you ever think of yourself as inferior, maybe because you're LGBTQ?
   - Are you hyper-vigilant? That is, are you always on the lookout for rejection or for things going wrong?
   - Do you find that your self-worth is dependent on how well you perform in certain parts of your life, like your appearance, your job, or being the best at various tasks?

- Do you frequently blame yourself for problems that go wrong in your life?
- Do you beat yourself up for feeling certain ways, or do you give yourself a hard time for getting upset about something?
- When you start to feel nervous, do you often worry it's going to increase into even more anxiety?
- When you start to feel down, do you feel like it's going to ruin your whole day?

3. What is your **Affect** (emotional experience) like when you are in situations that trigger LGBTQ-related stress?
   - Does it seem like you feel sad/anxious/frustrated more than other people?
   - Is it hard for you to stop thinking about things that upset, anger, or embarrass you?
   - Do you consider yourself a worrier?
   - Do you have trouble controlling your temper?
   - Have other people observed that your emotions seem more intense than others in response to situations?
   - Does it take you longer than other people to calm down when you get upset?
   - Does it seem like you feel things more intensely than other people?
   - How do you feel when you think of yourself and other LGBTQ people as inferior or negative?
   - How do you feel when you have identity-affirming thoughts of yourself as a proud, competent LGBTQ person?

4. What are your **Intentions** in these stressful situations?
   - Research finds that, in general, LGBTQ people are less optimistic than heterosexual, cisgender people with respect to believing that they will be able to live out their life dreams, hopes, and goals. Research also finds that LGBTQ people have a harder time on average asking for what they want or need in challenging situations. Is this true for you in the situations that you've identified as being challenging for you?
   - What do you want in these challenging situations? How do you want to feel, think, and behave?
   - What do you want in these situations that you might currently hold back from saying or doing?
   - What values guide your life? How are you acting out those values? How might you be holding back from living in

accordance with those values in challenging situations in your life?

5. What are your **Responses** to these challenging situations?
   - Do you tend to avoid or put off doing things that make you anxious?
   - Do you tend to avoid situations where you think you'll be uncomfortable?
   - Do you avoid doing things when you're in a bad mood or feeling down?
   - Do you try not to think about the things that make you upset?
   - Do you sometimes cope with uncomfortable emotions by trying to ignore them?
   - Are there things you wish you could do but don't because you're concerned about feeling a strong emotion, like anxiety, sadness, or frustration?
   - Do you try to do things to get rid of your negative emotions?
   - Do you try to do things to prevent yourself from feeling certain emotions?

6. What are the short-term and long-term **Consequences** of your responses to these challenging situations?
   - What do you think are the consequences of your response to these stressful situations? What happens after your response? Do you feel better in the short term? What about in the long term?
   - How has this strategy been working for you?
   - How does this strategy allow you to live as a thriving LGBTQ person?

7. What is your **Self-Evaluation** in these situations?
   - What is your current evaluation of yourself in challenging situations?
   - How would you like to evaluate yourself in these situations?

Preview of LGBTQ-Affirmative CBT

The chapters in this workbook program will address each component of the STAIRCaSE that you just started building. Table 2.1 presents a quick preview of what's to come, and how it will address your concerns.

Table 2.1. Preview of LGBTQ-Affirmative CBT

Chapter 3: Learning to Record Your Experiences	This chapter helps you start tracking your **Affect,** or emotions.
Chapter 4: Module 1: Setting Goals and Building Motivation for LGBTQ-Affirmative Cognitive-Behavioral Therapy	This chapter reviews what your **Intentions** are in situations that bring on LGBTQ-related stress.
Chapter 5: Module 2: Understanding the Nature and Emotional Impact of LGBTQ-Related Stress	This chapter explores the specific **Situations** that bring on LGBTQ-related stress.
Chapter 6: Module 3: Understanding and Tracking LGBTQ-Related Stress and Emotional Experiences	This chapter keeps exploring these stressful **Situations,** as well as the **Affect** (emotional experiences) you have in these situations
Chapter 7: Module 4: Increasing Mindful Awareness of LGBTQ-Related Stress Reactions	This chapter helps you develop skills for being aware of and nonjudgmental of your **Affect** in situations that bring up LGBTQ-related stress.
Chapter 8: Module 5: Increasing Cognitive Flexibility	This chapter will focus on skills to challenge unhelpful **Thoughts** you may have in situations that bring up LGBTQ-related stress, and to help you think in more flexible, helpful ways.
Chapter 9: Module 6: Countering Emotional Behaviors	This chapter will help you examine your **Responses** to stressful situations, and consider new, more helpful, ways of responding.
Chapter 10: Module 7: Experimenting with New Reactions to LGBTQ-Related Stress	This chapter teaches skills that cut across the entire STAIRCaSE. You'll purposefully enter stressful situations and use the skills that you've worked on in all the prior chapters to achieve your goals. You might experience new **Consequences** and **Self-Evaluation** from using these skills.
Chapter 11: Module 8: Emotion Exposures for Countering LGBTQ-Related Stress	In this chapter, you'll keep building up all your skills as you continue entering **Situations** that bring on strong **Affect**.
Chapter 12: Module 9: Recognizing Accomplishments and Looking to the Future	Wrapping up treatment, you'll have the opportunity to further clarify your **Intentions** in future challenging situations and continue looking for opportunities to strengthen your **Self-Evaluation** in the face of stress.

Home Practice: STAIRCaSE: Identifying When You Have Strong Emotions

Over the next week, spend some time thinking about the questions above to help you fill out Worksheet 2.1: The STAIRCaSE Model at the end of this chapter. Try to identify when and if you have strong emotions, and the thoughts that tend to accompany them. Describe the details of those thoughts the best you can.

But don't worry: Future chapters will teach you even more about how to think about your thinking. Future chapters will also help you identify those situations that might be contributing to your strong emotions and your typical responses in those situations. For now, try to identify the details of those situations and what you might do to try to avoid feeling strong emotions in those situations or perhaps avoid the situation altogether. What are the consequences of your reactions in those situations? And what is the impact that your behavior has on your self-evaluation? If you're working with a therapist, they will use this information to start to create a treatment plan for you. If not, that's okay—the treatment plan will come naturally as you move through the workbook.

Finally, be sure to try to identify your short- and long-term goals for yourself—Chapter 4 will help you do this even more. Figure 2.2 is an example of a completed STAIRCaSE Model worksheet.

Summary

In this chapter, you learned that emotions can be extremely distressing (and even considered emotional disorders) when they are characterized by frequent, intense, and negative reactions to emotions, including avoidance. Avoidance means avoiding the situation that might cause the emotion, or just trying to avoid feeling the emotion at all. You learned that LGBTQ-related stress can increase LGBTQ people's risk of emotional disorders in several ways, including by adding to general life stress, teaching LGBTQ people that their emotions are bad or wrong, and causing LGBTQ people to always be on the lookout for danger or rejection even in safe situations and relationships. The chapter finished by introducing the STAIRCaSE model as a way to prepare for the components of LGBTQ-affirmative CBT to be introduced in the remaining chapters of this workbook.

Worksheet 2.1: The STAIRCaSE Model

CHALLENGING **SITUATIONS**

THOUGHTS

STRONG UNCOMFORTABLE
EMOTIONS AND **AFFECT**

INTENTION (What do you want to do in this situation?)

AVOIDANT COPING **RESPONSES**

CONSEQUENCES
POSITIVE SHORT TERM:

NEGATIVE LONG TERM:

SELF-EVALUATION (How do
you currently view your behavior
in this situation?)

TREATMENT PLAN: FOCUS OF CORE MODULES
MODULE 4:
MODULE 5:
MODULE 6:
MODULE 7:
MODULE 8:

CHALLENGING SITUATIONS
- Anxiety when talking to new people
- Unhappy with social circle
- Difficulty expressing myself and asserting my needs in relationships

THOUGHTS
- Thinking that I've done something wrong
- Thinking that I'm not as good as other people
- Overthinking past "failures"
- "I need everyone to like me"

STRONG UNCOMFORTABLE EMOTIONS AND AFFECT
- Anxiety
- Shame
- Frustration and anger
- Upset stomach
- Tension

INTENTION (What do you want to do in this situation?)
I want to be able to be myself and express myself openly and authentically. I don't want to feel like I've done something wrong. I want to live according to my values.

AVOIDANT COPING RESPONSES
- Avoid social situations, dating
- Ruminating
- Not expressing myself and asserting my needs in relationships
- Avoiding difficult conversations
- Too much time on social media

CONSEQUENCES
POSITIVE SHORT TERM:
- I don't feel anxious when I avoid

NEGATIVE LONG TERM:
- I'm not living my best life, long-term anxiety

SELF-EVALUATION (How do you currently view your behavior in this situation?)
- I'm not the type of person who can socialize normally.
- I'm not the type of person who can express themselves.

TREATMENT PLAN: FOCUS OF CORE MODULES
MODULE 4: Practice nonjudgment about having few friends; anchor in the present when anxious
MODULE 5: Reframe likelihood of being rejected; let go of internalized shame rooted LGBTQ-related stress
MODULE 6: Identify LGBTQ-related stress source of avoidant coping; generate alternate actions
MODULE 7: Express my genuine opinions and beliefs; stay in safe social situations
MODULE 8: Exposure to blushing, exposure to jitteriness, exposure to physical tension

Figure 2.2

Example of a Completed STAIRCaSE Model Worksheet

CHAPTER 3 — Learning to Record Your Experiences

Chapter 3 Overview

In this chapter, you'll learn about the importance of recording your symptoms of anxiety and depression. You will learn how this can give you an objective, "scientific" view of your symptoms and inform your progress throughout this treatment.

Chapter 3 Outline

- The Importance of Record-Keeping
- Becoming an Objective Observer
- Learning How to Track Your Progress Throughout This Program
- Summary
- Home Practice: Starting to Record Your Emotions

The Importance of Record-Keeping

Throughout the course of this treatment program, you will be asked to complete a weekly questionnaire about your symptoms of anxiety and depression. These forms are located at the end of each chapter in the book. You may also download copies by searching for this book's title on the Oxford Academic platform at academic.oup.com.

There are many reasons why it is important to keep records of your experiences on a regular basis. First, intense anxiety, sadness, or other uncomfortable emotions typically feel overwhelming. Learning to be an observer of your own emotions is a first step towards understanding these experiences and feeling more in control. Throughout this treatment, you will learn specific skills that will help you respond to your emotions in more helpful ways. As you practice applying your new skills, ongoing monitoring will highlight the impact they are having on your emotional experiences. You'll be able to answer the question, "How is this new strategy helping?" Finally, monitoring your overall progress during the treatment (using the Progress Record) will help you track the gains you are making.

Monitoring your emotional experiences each week provides much more accurate information than simply asking yourself, "How have I been feeling lately?" If you were asked to describe the past week, you may judge it to have been very bad even though you felt relatively good at some points. Or you might evaluate how you felt over the entire week on the basis of how you felt over just the past couple of days. Focusing on your negative emotions makes it easy to forget about the times you didn't feel that way. Not only that, these negative judgments about how you've been doing in general may be contributing to your ongoing feelings of anxiety, sadness, or other distressing emotions. Keeping weekly records of your emotional experiences helps you to recognize that your mood fluctuates throughout the day and the week. Through this process, you will begin to get a more realistic picture of what is really going on for you, enabling you to feel more in control.

Becoming an Objective Observer

Sometimes people are concerned that continually recording how they're feeling will make them feel even worse. It is important to realize, however, that the way you observe your experiences matters. For example, **subjective monitoring** might mean focusing on how bad you feel, how much your emotions are interfering in your life, and how helpless you feel to control them.

In contrast, we'll be asking you to engage in **objective monitoring**, which involves observing your emotions in a more "scientific" way. In this program, you will learn to record things such as how many times over the course of the week you felt a certain way, what was happening right before you felt distressed, and how you responded (what you were thinking, doing, and feeling). In other words, you will be recording just the facts and evidence, not your judgments or evaluations of how good or bad the experience may have been for you.

At first, it may be difficult to switch from subjective to objective monitoring. As you start to use the record forms included in this workbook, you may even notice an increase in your distress because you are focusing on your emotions in the old, subjective way. However, with practice, you will begin to find switching into the objective mode easier and easier.

Learning How to Track Your Progress Throughout This Program

As you go through each chapter in this book, you will be introduced to specific record forms that have been developed to help you practice each new skill. In addition, there are two forms that you will use throughout the entire program. These forms will allow you to objectively record how often you experienced the general anxiety and depression common to all emotional disorders over the past week, as well as how much these feelings interfered with your daily life. These forms are called the Overall Depression Severity and Interference Scale (ODSIS)[1] (**Depression Scale**) and the Overall Anxiety Severity and Interference Scale (OASIS)[2] (**Anxiety Scale**). We will ask you to complete these two measures every week for the duration of your program.

[2]Use the information gathered from the Anxiety and Depression Scales (as well as the Other Assessment to track any other emotion-related behaviors you would like to track as part of your treatment goals) to chart your progress week by week on the **Progress Record**. The Progress Record

1   Bentley, K. H., Gallagher, M. W., Carl, J.R., & Barlow, D. H. (2014) Development and validation of the Overall Depression Severity and Impairment Scale. *Psychological Assessment, 26*, 815–830.

2   Norman, S. B., Cissell, S. H., Means-Christensen, A. J., & Stein, M. B. (2006). Development and validation of an Overall Anxiety Severity and Impairment Scale (OASIS). *Depression and Anxiety, 23*, 245–249.

is designed to summarize your improvement so that you can easily view changes over the course of the entire program. During each week of the program, you can indicate your score on the ODSIS and OASIS on the Progress Record. You can also use the Progress Record to record any additional emotion-related behaviors or symptoms you would like to address in this treatment. A blank copy of the Progress Record is provided at the end of this chapter and is also available to download by searching for this book's title on the Oxford Academic platform at academic.oup.com. On the bottom of the scale, you will see one section for each week you use this program. Use the numbers on the left side of the scale to plot your total score on the Anxiety and Depression Scales for each week. You may want to use a different-colored pen for each scale or a different shape to plot the score for each scale in order to tell the scales apart. If you are working through this program with a therapist, you might be asked to complete these scales at the start of each session, along with graphing your progress from week to week on the Progress Record.

You can also use the Progress Record to track any other behaviors you want to decrease (for example, drug or alcohol use) or increase (for example, standing up for your wants and needs or navigating a social situation you've been avoiding).

As you complete the weekly questionnaire, keep in mind that the goal of tracking your mood and anxiety is not to get "better" ratings each week. In fact, some of the practice skills in the treatment might bring up uncomfortable or negative emotions for you. The goal, instead, is to be more aware of how your mood and anxiety regularly fluctuate. In general, we expect that you will experience a *decrease* in anxiety, depression, and other emotional distress as you begin to practice the skills included in this treatment. As shown in Figure 3.1, progress does not occur in a straight line, but instead there are some peaks and valleys along the way. This is typical for most people. Oftentimes, people notice a spike in their anxiety and depression during times of increased stress. Additionally, people sometimes notice an increase in their distress as they start making hard and meaningful changes in their lives. In these cases, the increase in distress is a marker of really challenging oneself. If you find your own experience seems to be worse one week than it was the week before, challenge yourself to keep going. The goal of the treatment program is to have fewer of these "spikes" in distress. When they do occur, with practice, you'll be able to respond differently to them so that your emotional experiences are less intense and don't last as long.

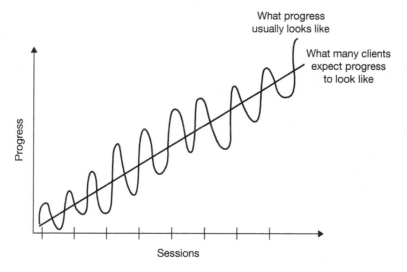

Figure 3.1

Progress in Treatment Does Not Always Follow a Straight Line
Figure created by Annette Yates.

Summary

We cannot emphasize enough the importance of record-keeping. Remember, there is a difference between *subjective* monitoring (focusing on how bad you feel) and *objective* monitoring (looking at the features of your experience in a more "scientific" way). Completing the **Anxiety** and **Depression Scales** and **Progress Record** weekly will help you keep your progress in perspective. At first, you may have to push yourself to complete these records, but it will become easier, and even rewarding, as you continue. These records not only serve to give yourself feedback but are also very helpful to your therapist, if you are working with one.

In the next chapter, we will present two more important concepts that will help prepare you to start this treatment program: setting your treatment goals and maintaining your motivation to engage in treatment.

Home Practice: Starting to Record Your Emotions

Try completing the forms labeled "ODSIS" and "OASIS" at the end of this chapter. Be sure to record your ODSIS and OASIS scores for this week on the Progress Record above "Week 1." Remember that you can also use the Progress Record to monitor any other emotion-driven behaviors or symptoms you would like to address during this treatment.

Overall Depression Severity and Interference Scale (ODSIS)

Instructions: The following items ask about depression. For each item, indicate the number for the answer that best describes your experience over the past week.

—1. In the past week, how often have you felt depressed?

    0 = **No depression** in the past week.

    1 = **Infrequent depression**. Felt depressed a few times.

    2 = **Occasional depression**. Felt depressed as much of the time as not.

    3 = **Frequent depression**. Felt depressed most of the time.

    4 = **Constant depression**. Felt depressed all of the time.

—2. In the past week, when you have felt depressed, how intense or severe was your depression?

    0 = **Little or None**: Depression was absent or barely noticeable.

    1 = **Mild**: Depression was at a low level.

    2 = **Moderate**: Depression was intense at times.

    3 = **Severe**: Depression was intense much of the time.

    4 = **Extreme**: Depression was overwhelming.

—3. In the past week, how often did you have difficulty engaging in or being interested in activities you normally enjoy because of depression?

    0 = **None**: I had no difficulty engaging in or being interested in activities that I normally enjoy because of depression.

    1 = **Infrequent**: A few times I had difficulty engaging in or being interested in activities that I normally enjoy because of depression. My lifestyle was not affected.

    2 = **Occasional**: I had some difficulty engaging in or being interested in activities that I normally enjoy because of depression. My lifestyle has only changed in minor ways.

    3 = **Frequent**: I have considerable difficulty engaging in or being interested in activities that I normally enjoy because of depression. I have made significant changes in my lifestyle because of being unable to become interested in activities I used to enjoy.

    4 = **All the Time**: I have been unable to participate in or be interested in activities that I normally enjoy because of depression. My lifestyle has been extensively affected and I no longer do things that I used to enjoy.

—4. In the past week, how much did your depression interfere with your ability to do the things you needed to do at work, at school, or at home?

    0 = **None**: No interference at work/home/school from depression.

    1 = **Mild**: My depression has caused some interference at work/home/school. Things are more difficult, but everything that needs to be done is still getting done.

    2 = **Moderate**: My depression definitely interferes with tasks. Most things are still getting done, but few things are being done as well as in the past.

    3 = **Severe**: My depression has really changed my ability to get things done. Some tasks are still being done, but many things are not. My performance has definitely suffered.

4 = **Extreme**: My depression has become incapacitating. I am unable to complete tasks and have had to leave school, have quit or been fired from my job, or have been unable to complete tasks at home and have faced consequences like bill collectors, eviction, etc.

—5. In the past week, how much has depression interfered with your social life and relationships?

0 = **None**: My depression doesn't affect my relationships.

1 = **Mild**: My depression slightly interferes with my relationships. Some of my friendships and other relationships have suffered, but, overall, my social life is still fulfilling.

2 = **Moderate**: I have experienced some interference with my social life, but I still have a few close relationships. I don't spend as much time with others as in the past, but I still socialize sometimes.

3 = **Severe**: My friendships and other relationships have suffered a lot because of depression. I do not enjoy social activities. I socialize very little.

4 = **Extreme**: My depression has completely disrupted my social activities. All of my relationships have suffered or ended. My family life is extremely strained.

Total Score: ___

Overall Anxiety Severity and Interference Scale (OASIS)

Instructions: The following items ask about anxiety and fear. For each item, indicate the number for the answer that best describes your experience over the past week.

—1. In the past week, how often have you felt anxious?

    0 = **No anxiety** in the past week.

    1 = **Infrequent anxiety.** Felt anxious a few times.

    2 = **Occasional anxiety.** Felt anxious as much of the time as not. It was hard to relax.

    3 = **Frequent anxiety.** Felt anxious most of the time. It was very difficult to relax.

    4 = **Constant anxiety.** Felt anxious all of the time and never really relaxed.

—2. In the past week, when you have felt anxious, how intense or severe was your anxiety?

    0 = **Little or None:** Anxiety was absent or barely noticeable.

    1 = **Mild:** Anxiety was at a low level. It was possible to relax when I tried. Physical symptoms were only slightly uncomfortable.

    2 = **Moderate:** Anxiety was distressing at times. It was hard to relax or concentrate, but I could do it if I tried. Physical symptoms were uncomfortable.

    3 = **Severe:** Anxiety was intense much of the time. It was very difficult to relax or focus on anything else. Physical symptoms were extremely uncomfortable.

    4 = **Extreme:** Anxiety was overwhelming. It was impossible to relax at all. Physical symptoms were unbearable.

—3. In the past week, how often did you avoid situations, places, objects, or activities because of anxiety or fear?

    0 = **None:** I do not avoid places, situations, activities, or things because of fear.

    1 = **Infrequent:** I avoid something once in a while, but will usually face the situation or confront the object. My lifestyle is not affected.

    2 = **Occasional:** I have some fear of certain situations, places, or objects, but it is still manageable. My lifestyle has only changed in minor ways. I always or almost always avoid the things I fear when I'm alone, but can handle them if someone comes with me.

    3 = **Frequent:** I have considerable fear and really try to avoid the things that frighten me. I have made significant changes in my lifestyle to avoid the object, situation, activity, or place.

    4 = **All the Time:** Avoiding objects, situations, activities, or places has taken over my life. My lifestyle has been extensively affected and I no longer do things that I used to enjoy.

—4. In the past week, how much did your anxiety interfere with your ability to do the things you needed to do at work, at school, or at home?

    0 = **None:** No interference at work/home/school from anxiety.

    1 = **Mild:** My anxiety has caused some interference at work/home/school. Things are more difficult, but everything that needs to be done is still getting done.

2 = **Moderate:** My anxiety definitely interferes with tasks. Most things are still getting done, but few things are being done as well as in the past.

3 = **Severe:** My anxiety has really changed my ability to get things done. Some tasks are still being done, but many things are not. My performance has definitely suffered.

4 = **Extreme:** My anxiety has become incapacitating. I am unable to complete tasks and have had to leave school, have quit or been fired from my job, or have been unable to complete tasks at home and have faced consequences like bill collectors, eviction, etc.

—5. In the past week, how much has anxiety interfered with your social life and relationships?

0 = **None:** My anxiety doesn't affect my relationships.

1 = **Mild:** My anxiety slightly interferes with my relationships. Some of my friendships and other relationships have suffered, but, overall, my social life is still fulfilling.

2 = **Moderate:** I have experienced some interference with my social life, but I still have a few close relationships. I don't spend as much time with others as in the past, but I still socialize sometimes.

3 = **Severe:** My friendships and other relationships have suffered a lot because of anxiety. I do not enjoy social activities. I socialize very little.

4 = **Extreme:** My anxiety has completely disrupted my social activities. All of my relationships have suffered or ended. My family life is extremely strained.

Total Score: ____

Progress Record

ODSIS

```
20 ——————————————————————————————
18 ——————————————————————————————
16 ——————————————————————————————
14 ——————————————————————————————
12 ——————————————————————————————
10 ——————————————————————————————
 8 ——————————————————————————————
 6 ——————————————————————————————
 4 ——————————————————————————————
 2 ——————————————————————————————
 0 ——————————————————————————————
```

| Week | 1 | 2 | 3 | 4 | 5 | 6 | 7 | 8 | 9 | 10 | 11 | 12 | 13 | 14 | 15 | 16 | 17 | 18 | 19 | 20 | 21 | 22 | 23 | 24 | v |

OASIS

```
20 ——————————————————————————————
18 ——————————————————————————————
16 ——————————————————————————————
14 ——————————————————————————————
12 ——————————————————————————————
10 ——————————————————————————————
 8 ——————————————————————————————
 6 ——————————————————————————————
 4 ——————————————————————————————
 2 ——————————————————————————————
 0 ——————————————————————————————
```

| Week | 1 | 2 | 3 | 4 | 5 | 6 | 7 | 8 | 9 | 10 | 11 | 12 | 13 | 14 | 15 | 16 | 17 | 18 | 19 | 20 | 21 | 22 | 23 | 24 | v |

Other Assessment

```
20 ——————————————————————————————
18 ——————————————————————————————
16 ——————————————————————————————
14 ——————————————————————————————
12 ——————————————————————————————
10 ——————————————————————————————
 8 ——————————————————————————————
 6 ——————————————————————————————
 4 ——————————————————————————————
 2 ——————————————————————————————
 0 ——————————————————————————————
```

| Week | 1 | 2 | 3 | 4 | 5 | 6 | 7 | 8 | 9 | 10 | 11 | 12 | 13 | 14 | 15 | 16 | 17 | 18 | 19 | 20 | 21 | 22 | 23 | 24 | v |

Module 1: Setting Goals and Building Motivation for LGBTQ-Affirmative Cognitive-Behavioral Therapy

Chapter 4 Overview

In this chapter, you'll read about the importance of building motivation and setting goals so that you can get the most out of this program. You'll start by thinking about your motivations for engaging in behavioral health care, as well as the pros and cons of making changes to your life. Then, you'll think about your goals for treatment.

Chapter 4 Outline

- Weekly Check-In
- Motivation: Change Starts with You!
- The Pros and Cons of Changing
- Goal Setting: What Do YOU Want to Change?
- Summary
- Home Practice: Setting Treatment Goals

Weekly Check-In

In the last chapter, you learned about "progress monitoring"—that is, completing questionnaires regarding your symptoms of anxiety, depression, and any other symptoms that may be important for you to keep track of. We have a new copy of those questionnaires at the end of this chapter (labeled "ODSIS" and "OASIS"). You may also photocopy these forms or download multiple copies by searching for this book's title on the Oxford Academic platform at academic.oup.com. Take a moment to complete those now. Remember, you have your Progress Record that you can use to track your symptoms over time, which is located at the end of Chapter 3.

It's still very early in treatment, but you may be able to see how your symptoms are changing even at this early stage of the treatment. Keep in mind that progress does not go in a straight line—it's normal to see ups and downs in your symptoms.

Motivation: Change Starts with You!

People who seek this treatment often hope to improve the way they feel, stop behaving in unhelpful ways, and generally improve their life. Research shows that two factors strongly affect how much they end up benefiting from therapy:

1. How much a person engages in the treatment (completing all outside-of-session work, doing all the exercises, challenging themselves to face uncomfortable situations to make things better); and
2. How motivated and committed a person is to changing.

Knowing how important these factors are for getting the most out of therapy, we have developed some ways to help keep you motivated throughout treatment.

Keep in Mind That Motivation Is Not Fixed

It changes over time. Some days your motivation will be high and completing all the activities that are part of this treatment program will be pretty easy. On other days it might be more difficult to get yourself to read the chapter or complete the home practice activities. Feeling stressed at school, work, or home, or feeling tired or sick, can make it hard to stay motivated. At some points, you might even feel like you don't want to change, or like it's not worth the time and effort. This is a normal, natural part of the change process. It's important to let yourself have these moments. Those hard days are also when it can be even the most useful to push yourself to engage with this treatment program—including completing the chapters and the home practice exercises.

You're in Control

In Chapter 2, you learned about the concept of LGBTQ-related stress. One lesson that LGBTQ-related stress can falsely have LGBTQ people believe is that they are not in control—of themselves, their relationships, or their emotions—and that their decisions and life options are set by other people, not themselves. In this treatment, you're in control, and you get to decide how you want to use the tools you learn here to address the impact of stigma and LGBTQ-related stress in your life.

The Pros and Cons of Changing

When thinking about making a change, it's sometimes hard to see all sides. It's common to ignore things that you may not want to do or feel are too hard to do. Use Worksheet 4.1: Decisional Balance Worksheet to evaluate your choices and help you think through all the pros and cons of changing and not changing. A blank copy of the worksheet is provided at the end of this chapter and is also available to download by searching for this book's title on the Oxford Academic platform at academic.oup.com. Let's practice.

First, think of a behavior that you would like to change in the context of this treatment program (e.g., "I don't share my difficult feelings with other people"):

_____

Now, on Worksheet 4.1: Decisional Balance Worksheet, write down at least one pro and one con for making a change that you would like to make. Then write down at least one pro and one con for letting things stay the same. These pro/con statements can be as big or small, as specific or general, as you would like. Just begin by writing one in each box on the worksheet.

Table 4.2, on page 46, shows an example of how the Decisional Balance Worksheet might be completed by someone who has the goal of talking to people after class in order to make friends.

You can also complete the Decisional Balance Worksheet by thinking more generally about what you see as the pros and cons of engaging in this treatment program (and making the changes to your life associated with that) versus not engaging in treatment (and continuing to stay the same).

Goal Setting: What Do You Want to Change?

One of the most effective ways to change your behavior is through goal setting. Goals can include big-picture things, like "being more content," or more specific things, like "seeing my friend more regularly." Achieving a goal requires changing a behavior to help accomplish that goal. Table 4.1 shows a list of problem behaviors that are commonly faced by LGBTQ individuals because of LGBTQ-related stress. Perhaps you're experiencing some of these behaviors, or perhaps you're experiencing other types of problems.

Now that you've seen some examples of problems that other LGBTQ people often experience, try writing out some of your own using Worksheet 4.2: Treatment Goals and Examples, which is located at the end of the chapter. You may also download a copy by searching for this book's title on the Oxford Academic platform at academic.oup.com. Under "Problems," describe a few of your problems. Then, under "Examples," write down a specific example of how each problem has recently impacted you. Don't worry if the problem seems similar (or not) to the examples above. The important thing is to choose something you'd like to work on during this treatment program.

In future chapters, you'll learn that many of these problems are driven by emotions. You'll also learn to use tools to help make these emotions feel more manageable (although it might be hard to believe that right now). You can get there as long as you have a clear goal that can be broken down into steps. This might sound like a lot. Don't worry! You can take it one step at a time to help you meet your goals.

Now, take a look at Worksheet 4.3: Treatment Goal Setting Worksheet, which is located at the end of the chapter. You may also download a copy by searching for this book's title on the Oxford Academic platform at academic.oup.com. Use this worksheet as an opportunity to think about your goals for this treatment program in more detail. If you are working

Table 4.1. Problems Commonly Faced by LGBTQ Clients

Problem	Example
Avoiding romantic connections with people of the same gender	Patrick has sex with other men and wants to have a deeper relationship with one of his partners, but avoids asking him on a date because he fears it will make him "gayer."
Being a perfectionist at school, work, or home	Sarah spends 2 minutes writing but 40 minutes editing an email to a friend because she is afraid of what her friend will think.
Avoiding heterosexual or cisgender people	Alex has a career that requires networking, but they avoid going to work social events because most of their coworkers are straight and cisgender.
Being closeted	Dakota has known that he is attracted to people of all genders for many years but has not shared that important part of himself with any other people, including his spouse.
Escaping social situations	Dominique arrives early to a party and only stays to chat with the host, but feels anxious and leaves when other guests start to arrive.
Not expressing your needs, opinions, preferences	Laura goes with her friend to events that she strongly prefers not to attend, but doesn't say anything because she doesn't want to upset her friend.
Relying on alcohol or drugs to control your mood	Brent feels anxious about meeting other men for sex, and always has two beers and a joint to "take the edge off" before hooking up with someone.
Withdrawing from others completely	Sasha feels so down that they say no to invitations to go out, don't respond to texts, and never check their emails.
Aggression towards others	Max's temper and hurtful remarks always seem to burn bridges with the people they care most about.
Constantly worrying about being rejected by others	When in public, Fiona constantly monitors whether people are looking or laughing at her or her girlfriend.
Avoiding talking to a doctor about sexual health	Ricardo doesn't know his HIV status, but is afraid to talk about sex with his partners or his doctor.
Avoiding gay spaces	Marcus feels that his body is not where he would want it to be physically, and feels self-conscious about his looks. He therefore avoids going to gay venues, avoids starting conversations with other gay men, and has a hard time dating and forming romantic relationships.

with a therapist, they might work with you to set all three treatment goals, or they might have you complete one goal in the session and the rest for home practice. If you're working on your own, complete this worksheet at your own pace. Box 4.1, on page 51, is an example of a completed Treatment Goal Setting Worksheet.

Below are a few things to remember while you complete your Treatment Goal Setting Worksheet.

Set Specific Goals

For example, setting the goal of "Get more LGBTQ friends" isn't an ideal goal because it doesn't tell you how to get more friends—or what that would even look like! Do you want lots of LGBTQ online friends who you follow on social media but never see in person? Or, do you want two or three new LGBTQ friends who you see in person most weeks? You would approach these two goals in very different ways. Examples of more specific goals are:

- "I would see LGBTQ friends at least a few times per week."
- "I would spend more time with other people, rather than being by myself all the time."
- "I would try to approach new people I meet, instead of avoiding people."

Develop Steps Toward Each Goal

Once you have a specific and concrete overall goal, try breaking it down into smaller steps that will help you get there. To do this, you can try asking yourself:

- "What would I be doing that I'm not currently doing if I was closer to my goal?"
- "What would it look like for me to be living my daily life in a way that is consistent with my goal?"

Remember: This Is an Exercise

Completing your Treatment Goal Setting Worksheet is a practice exercise, and it may feel hard to do! If you feel stuck, take some time to look back at the examples shown earlier and think about what first motivated you to seek treatment. If you're working with a therapist, you can also let them know that you're feeling stuck. Feel free to take breaks. Working through the exercise completely is more important than doing it "perfectly."

Summary

In this chapter, you started thinking in more detail about your motivation for engaging in this treatment—as well as any downsides of engaging in treatment. It's normal to experience highs and lows in motivation; the reasons for changing that you identified in this chapter and the downsides of staying the same that you identified can help your motivation for treatment. You also started thinking about your goals for treatment. Thinking about your goals is another great way to stay motivated!

Home Practice: Setting Treatment Goals

Before going on to the next chapter, be sure to complete Worksheet 4.3: Treatment Goal Setting Worksheet to set clear goals for your treatment. Remember, this is "practice"—just like with sports, school, or hobbies, we only get better by practicing often. If you find that you feel frustrated, that's okay. Practice can be hard sometimes! As progress happens over time, there are sometimes setbacks and sometimes improvements. Feel free to take a break. Try doing the home practice activities on different days or at different times until you find out what works best for you.

Overall Depression Severity and Interference Scale (ODSIS)

Instructions: The following items ask about depression. For each item, indicate the number for the answer that best describes your experience over the past week.

—1. In the past week, how often have you felt depressed?

0 = **No depression** in the past week.

1 = **Infrequent depression**. Felt depressed a few times.

2 = **Occasional depression**. Felt depressed as much of the time as not.

3 = **Frequent depression**. Felt depressed most of the time.

4 = **Constant depression**. Felt depressed all of the time.

—2. In the past week, when you have felt depressed, how intense or severe was your depression?

0 = **Little or None**: Depression was absent or barely noticeable.

1 = **Mild**: Depression was at a low level.

2 = **Moderate**: Depression was intense at times.

3 = **Severe**: Depression was intense much of the time.

4 = **Extreme**: Depression was overwhelming.

—3. In the past week, how often did you have difficulty engaging in or being interested in activities you normally enjoy because of depression?

0 = **None**: I had no difficulty engaging in or being interested in activities that I normally enjoy because of depression.

1 = **Infrequent**: A few times I had difficulty engaging in or being interested in activities that I normally enjoy because of depression. My lifestyle was not affected.

2 = **Occasional**: I had some difficulty engaging in or being interested in activities that I normally enjoy because of depression. My lifestyle has only changed in minor ways.

3 = **Frequent**: I have considerable difficulty engaging in or being interested in activities that I normally enjoy because of depression. I have made significant changes in my lifestyle because of being unable to become interested in activities I used to enjoy.

4 = **All the Time**: I have been unable to participate in or be interested in activities that I normally enjoy because of depression. My lifestyle has been extensively affected and I no longer do things that I used to enjoy.

—4. In the past week, how much did your depression interfere with your ability to do the things you needed to do at work, at school, or at home?

0 = **None**: No interference at work/home/school from depression.

1 = **Mild**: My depression has caused some interference at work/home/school. Things are more difficult, but everything that needs to be done is still getting done.

2 = **Moderate**: My depression definitely interferes with tasks. Most things are still getting done, but few things are being done as well as in the past.

3 = **Severe**: My depression has really changed my ability to get things done. Some tasks are still being done, but many things are not. My performance has definitely suffered.

4 = **Extreme**: My depression has become incapacitating. I am unable to complete tasks and have had to leave school, have quit or been fired from my job, or have been unable to complete tasks at home and have faced consequences like bill collectors, eviction, etc.

—5. In the past week, how much has depression interfered with your social life and relationships?

0 = **None**: My depression doesn't affect my relationships.

1 = **Mild**: My depression slightly interferes with my relationships. Some of my friendships and other relationships have suffered, but, overall, my social life is still fulfilling.

2 = **Moderate**: I have experienced some interference with my social life, but I still have a few close relationships. I don't spend as much time with others as in the past, but I still socialize sometimes.

3 = **Severe**: My friendships and other relationships have suffered a lot because of depression. I do not enjoy social activities. I socialize very little.

4 = **Extreme**: My depression has completely disrupted my social activities. All of my relationships have suffered or ended. My family life is extremely strained.

Total Score: ___

Overall Anxiety Severity and Interference Scale (OASIS)

Instructions: The following items ask about anxiety and fear. For each item, indicate the number for the answer that best describes your experience over the past week.

—1. In the past week, how often have you felt anxious?

    0 = **No anxiety** in the past week.

    1 = **Infrequent anxiety.** Felt anxious a few times.

    2 = **Occasional anxiety.** Felt anxious as much of the time as not. It was hard to relax.

    3 = **Frequent anxiety.** Felt anxious most of the time. It was very difficult to relax.

    4 = **Constant anxiety.** Felt anxious all of the time and never really relaxed.

—2. In the past week, when you have felt anxious, how intense or severe was your anxiety?

    0 = **Little or None:** Anxiety was absent or barely noticeable.

    1 = **Mild:** Anxiety was at a low level. It was possible to relax when I tried. Physical symptoms were only slightly uncomfortable.

    2 = **Moderate:** Anxiety was distressing at times. It was hard to relax or concentrate, but I could do it if I tried. Physical symptoms were uncomfortable.

    3 = **Severe:** Anxiety was intense much of the time. It was very difficult to relax or focus on anything else. Physical symptoms were extremely uncomfortable.

    4 = **Extreme:** Anxiety was overwhelming. It was impossible to relax at all. Physical symptoms were unbearable.

—3. In the past week, how often did you avoid situations, places, objects, or activities because of anxiety or fear?

    0 = **None:** I do not avoid places, situations, activities, or things because of fear.

    1 = **Infrequent:** I avoid something once in a while, but will usually face the situation or confront the object. My lifestyle is not affected.

    2 = **Occasional:** I have some fear of certain situations, places, or objects, but it is still manageable. My lifestyle has only changed in minor ways. I always or almost always avoid the things I fear when I'm alone, but can handle them if someone comes with me.

    3 = **Frequent:** I have considerable fear and really try to avoid the things that frighten me. I have made significant changes in my lifestyle to avoid the object, situation, activity, or place.

    4 = **All the Time:** Avoiding objects, situations, activities, or places has taken over my life. My lifestyle has been extensively affected and I no longer do things that I used to enjoy.

—4. In the past week, how much did your anxiety interfere with your ability to do the things you needed to do at work, at school, or at home?

    0 = **None:** No interference at work/home/school from anxiety.

    1 = **Mild:** My anxiety has caused some interference at work/home/school. Things are more difficult, but everything that needs to be done is still getting done.

2 = **Moderate:** My anxiety definitely interferes with tasks. Most things are still getting done, but few things are being done as well as in the past.

3 = **Severe:** My anxiety has really changed my ability to get things done. Some tasks are still being done, but many things are not. My performance has definitely suffered.

4 = **Extreme:** My anxiety has become incapacitating. I am unable to complete tasks and have had to leave school, have quit or been fired from my job, or have been unable to complete tasks at home and have faced consequences like bill collectors, eviction, etc.

—5. In the past week, how much has anxiety interfered with your social life and relationships?

0 = **None:** My anxiety doesn't affect my relationships.

1 = **Mild:** My anxiety slightly interferes with my relationships. Some of my friendships and other relationships have suffered, but, overall, my social life is still fulfilling.

2 = **Moderate:** I have experienced some interference with my social life, but I still have a few close relationships. I don't spend as much time with others as in the past, but I still socialize sometimes.

3 = **Severe:** My friendships and other relationships have suffered a lot because of anxiety. I do not enjoy social activities. I socialize very little.

4 = **Extreme:** My anxiety has completely disrupted my social activities. All of my relationships have suffered or ended. My family life is extremely strained.

Total Score: ___

Progress Record

ODSIS

```
20 ────────────────────────────────────
18 ────────────────────────────────────
16 ────────────────────────────────────
14 ────────────────────────────────────
12 ────────────────────────────────────
10 ────────────────────────────────────
 8 ────────────────────────────────────
 6 ────────────────────────────────────
 4 ────────────────────────────────────
 2 ────────────────────────────────────
 0 ────────────────────────────────────
```

Week 1 2 3 4 5 6 7 8 9 10 11 12 13 14 15 16 17 18 19 20 21 22 23 24 v

OASIS

```
20 ────────────────────────────────────
18 ────────────────────────────────────
16 ────────────────────────────────────
14 ────────────────────────────────────
12 ────────────────────────────────────
10 ────────────────────────────────────
 8 ────────────────────────────────────
 6 ────────────────────────────────────
 4 ────────────────────────────────────
 2 ────────────────────────────────────
 0 ────────────────────────────────────
```

Week 1 2 3 4 5 6 7 8 9 10 11 12 13 14 15 16 17 18 19 20 21 22 23 24 v

Other Assessment

```
20 ────────────────────────────────────
18 ────────────────────────────────────
16 ────────────────────────────────────
14 ────────────────────────────────────
12 ────────────────────────────────────
10 ────────────────────────────────────
 8 ────────────────────────────────────
 6 ────────────────────────────────────
 4 ────────────────────────────────────
 2 ────────────────────────────────────
 0 ────────────────────────────────────
```

Week 1 2 3 4 5 6 7 8 9 10 11 12 13 14 15 16 17 18 19 20 21 22 23 24 v

Worksheet 4.1: Decisional Balance Worksheet

	Pros/Benefits	Cons/Costs
Change		
Stay the Same		

Table 4.2. Example Decisional Balance Worksheet

	Pros/Benefits	Cons/Costs
Change	I could receive support and maybe new perspectives on the difficulties I face.	It would be hard and scary to open up about my emotions; I might get rejected.
Stay the Same	I don't have to do anything different; things are comfortable the way they are; I can stay in my comfort zone.	I would keep thinking about my difficulties over and over again and feel alone.

Worksheet 4.2: Treatment Goals and Examples

Problems	Examples
1.	
2.	
3.	

Worksheet 4.3: Treatment Goal Setting Worksheet

My #1 goal for treatment is:

_____

Making It More Concrete

Now, let's take a moment to make this goal more concrete. What would your life look like once you have achieved this goal? What things would you be doing, or not doing? What behaviors would you be engaging in? What behaviors would you *not* be engaging in? Try to be as concrete as possible here.

_____

_____

_____

_____

Taking the Necessary Steps

Next, think about some small manageable steps that you can take towards reaching the specific treatment goals you've listed above. These steps should take anywhere from a few days, a week, or up to a month to achieve. What steps will you need to take? Use the behaviors you listed above to help come up with your steps to achieving your treatment goal.

Step 1:

_____

Step 2:

_____

Step 3:

_____

Step 4:

_____

Step 5:

_____

People often have at least a few goals for treatment. Let's take a moment to list at least two more treatment goals you have. You might find it helpful to repeat this process for additional goals as well.

My #2 goal for treatment is:

_____

Making It More Concrete

Now, let's take a moment to make this goal more concrete. What would your life look like once you have achieved this goal? What things would you be doing, or not doing? What behaviors would you be engaging in? What behaviors would you *not* be engaging in? Try to be as concrete as possible here.

_____

_____

_____

_____

Taking the Necessary Steps

Next, think about some small manageable steps that you can take towards reaching the specific treatment goals you've listed above. These steps should take anywhere from a few days, a week, or up to a month to achieve. What steps will you need to take? Use the behaviors you listed above to help come up with your steps to achieving your treatment goal.

Step 1:

_____

Step 2:

_____

Step 3:

_____

Step 4:

_____

Step 5:

_____

My #3 goal for treatment is:

_____

Making It More Concrete

Now, let's take a moment to make this goal more concrete. What would your life look like once you have achieved this goal? What things would you be doing, or not doing? What behaviors would you be engaging in? What behaviors would you *not* be engaging in? Try to be as concrete as possible here.

_____

_____

_____

_____

Taking the Necessary Steps
Next, think about some small manageable steps that you can take towards reaching the specific treatment goals you've listed above. These steps should take anywhere from a few days, a week, or up to a month to achieve. What steps will you need to take? Use the behaviors you listed above to help come up with your steps to achieving your treatment goal.

Step 1:

_____

Step 2:

_____

Step 3:

_____

Step 4:

_____

Step 5:

_____

Box 4.1. Treatment Goal Setting Worksheet—Example Goal

My #1 goal for treatment is:

To make more LGBTQ friends

Making it More Concrete

Now, let's take a moment to make this goal more concrete. What would your life look like once you have achieved this goal? What things would you be doing, or not doing? What behaviors would you be engaging in? What behaviors would you *not* be engaging in? Try to be as concrete as possible here.

I would see LGBTQ friends at least a few times per week. I would spend more time with other people, rather than being by myself all the time. I would try to approach new people I meet, instead of avoiding people

Taking the Necessary Steps

Next, think about some small manageable steps that you can take towards reaching the specific treatment goals you've listed above. These steps should take anywhere from a few days, a week, or up to a month to achieve. What steps will you need to take? Use the behaviors you listed above to help come up with your steps to achieving your treatment goal.

Step 1: Google LGBTQ youth groups/centers in my area.

Step 2: Talk to my parents about getting bus money so that I can get to the center.

Step 3: Go to the center and try to have a conversation with one person.

Step 4: Join a recurring group at the center.

Step 5: After meeting new people, ask for their phone numbers and insta handles to plan get-togethers outside the center.

Module 2: Understanding the Nature and Emotional Impact of LGBTQ-Related Stress

Chapter 5 Overview

Today, you will continue learning how to cope with LGBTQ-related stressors. The main goal for today is to learn how to recognize your own experiences of LGBTQ-related stress, and how that stress may make your general stress worse.

Chapter 5 Outline

- Weekly Check-In
- Review Home Practice from Chapter 4
- What Is LGBTQ-Related Stress?
- How Does LGBTQ-Related Stress Affect You?
- Identifying How LGBTQ-Related Stress Influences Your Emotions and Behaviors
- Summary
- Home Practice: Monitoring LGBTQ-Related Stress

Weekly Check-In

Take a minute to track your symptoms using the ODSIS and OASIS, located at the end of this chapter. You may also photocopy these forms or download multiple copies by searching for this book's title on the Oxford

Academic platform at academic.oup.com. Do you notice any changes? What do you attribute these changes to?

Review Home Practice from Chapter 4

Last week, we learned that one of the most effective ways to make changes is through setting goals and breaking them down into clear, achievable steps.

In Table 2.1, you read a list of challenging behaviors that are commonly faced by LGBTQ individuals as a result of LGBTQ-related stress (e.g., avoiding dating, not expressing your needs). We then asked which behaviors you might like to change.

What behaviors did you identify? Feel free to go back to the previous chapter in order to remember the behaviors. Writing down these behaviors will help you set clear, achievable steps towards changing them.

| |
| |
| |

Are there other behaviors you would like to add to the list?

| |
| |
| |

Last week you also to monitored your weekly experiences of depression and anxiety by completing the ODSIS and OASIS. If you have not had the chance to complete these yet, please take a minute to do so.

- Are there any changes you're noticing related to depression and anxiety?
- Any changes you want to see happen?

In the coming weeks, we will help you identify the changes that you are making. We will also help you identify and overcome barriers to feeling better.

What Is LGBTQ-Related Stress?

In the last chapter, you started learning about LGBTQ-related stress. In this chapter, you will reflect on how LGBTQ-related stress may be affecting you in your daily life.

LGBTQ people face LGBTQ-related stress as a result of a lifetime of being treated differently and often worse than non-LGBTQ people. When these experiences build up over time, many LGBTQ folks may feel like they have less control over their life. They might also feel unsure about their future.

This looks different in different people. Some people might always be on the lookout for rejection. Others might feel pressured to hide parts of themselves, or feel ashamed of their identity, preferences, or behavior. Regardless of how it looks, LGBTQ-related stress tends to make anxiety, depression, and related behaviors (like problems with substances, sex, or eating) worse.

Take Sarah for example. Sarah identifies as a lesbian woman, and she works at the movie theater on the weekend. At school, other people make fun of her for being a tomboy. She hides her interest in sports so her classmates will stop making fun of her. At work, Sarah finds herself pretending to find the homophobic jokes her coworkers tell funny. She is afraid she will be left out or bullied if she calls them out on their jokes.

Or Matt. Matt is a bisexual man who works out at the gym every day. When he came out, Matt's weight was heavier than average. He was rejected and judged by other gay and bisexual men because of his weight. Matt works out to avoid being judged or disliked, rather than for his own enjoyment.

Take a look at Worksheet 5.1 at the end of this chapter for some other examples of LGBTQ-related stress. You may also download a copy of this worksheet by searching for this book's title on the Oxford Academic platform at academic.oup.com.

A lifetime of some or many of these stressors may lead to long-lasting feelings of shame, guilt, or self-consciousness. For example, you may have learned, from an early age, that your needs, desires, and behaviors are bad or abnormal—that they are something to be ashamed of. You might start to believe this message, and this can affect how you respond in many situations.

Being treated differently, unfairly, or harshly for being LGBTQ—openly or subtly—can produce uncomfortable emotions.

And sometimes, other stressors can come from the LGBTQ community itself, causing other difficult emotions. For instance, many LGBTQ folks (e.g., bisexual people, transgender people, women, people with lower income, people of color) often report feeling bias, invisibility, stereotypes, and discrimination within the LGBTQ community. These stressors can sometimes make LGBTQ individuals feel inferior, causing them to go to lengths to show superiority to others even within the LGBTQ community.

Experience with any of these stressors can cause you to feel uncomfortable emotions, like sadness, anxiety, guilt, or shame. Over time, these emotions may develop into what are called emotional disorders, such as generalized anxiety disorder, social anxiety disorder, obsessive-compulsive disorder, panic disorder, and depression.

Studies have shown that LGBTQ individuals are much more likely than non-LGBTQ people to have mood and anxiety disorders because of the stress they face related to their identity. For many LGBTQ people, LGBTQ-related stress seems to contribute to depression, anxiety, and unhealthy coping behaviors, like substance use and risky sex.

Identifying How LGBTQ-Related Stress Influences Your Emotions and Behaviors

The main goal of this chapter is for you to reflect on your own experiences of LGBTQ-related stress, and to think about how this stress may contribute to your emotions and behaviors—the things that brought you to seek help from this program. After learning to identify your own experiences of LGBTQ-related stress, some of your challenging emotions and behaviors might start to make more sense. Ultimately, learning to recognize causes of your negative feelings and thoughts makes it easier to cope with them!

To help you, let's first come up with some unique stressors that LGBTQ people commonly face. On the lines below, write down two examples of stressful situations that are only experienced by LGBTQ people. These can be examples from Worksheet 5.1 or any other examples that you've noticed.

1. _____

_____

_____

_____

2. _____

_____

_____

_____

The following questions may help you recall some of your past experiences with LGBTQ-related stress:

- How comfortable do you feel with your family? Was this different in the past? What about extended family?
- Are there important people in your life who do not know you are LGBTQ?
- Do you hide your gender or romantic experiences from important people in your life?
- Did you ever find yourself pretending to be straight or cis, or moving away from your partner, in an environment that felt unaccepting?
- Do you ever modify your gender expression to avoid being treated badly by others?
- Are there other experiences that you think your non-LGBTQ friends or coworkers do not have to face?

Let's think about *your own* experiences of LGBTQ-related stress. On the lines below, describe two specific situations (one current and one from the past) when you felt stigmatized, inferior, or uncomfortable due to your sexual orientation or gender identity.

1. Current situation:

_____

_____

_____

2. Past situation:

_____

_____

_____

Reflecting on these painful experiences is difficult. If you need to, feel free to take a break before you continue.

As research shows, these stressful situations may have a lasting impact on your emotional well-being. They affect LGBTQ folks at the time they occur, of course, but can also continue to cause lasting difficult emotions (e.g., shame, sadness, fear, or other negative emotions). Using Worksheet 5.2 located at the end of this chapter, how do you think the stressors you identified for yourself impact your emotions? You may also download a copy of this worksheet by searching for this book's title on the Oxford Academic platform at academic.oup.com.

How do you think LGBTQ-related stress may have contributed to those behaviors you said you wanted to change in the last chapter? How has LGBTQ-related stress contributed to your depression or anxiety? Write these answers on the lines below:

_____

_____

_____

_____

_____

In future chapters, you will see how some of these past and ongoing experiences with LGBTQ-related stress might contribute to your difficulties today.

An Important Note: During this chapter and this week's home practice, uncomfortable and sometimes painful emotions may arise. While this home practice exercise may bring up difficult memories or experiences, it is important to recognize your own strengths. As an LGBTQ person, you have overcome stressors that many other people will never have to face, and it's important to acknowledge your ability to do so. You are resilient! The next chapters will build on your resilience to help you face difficult emotions with new skills.

Summary

In this chapter, you continued to develop your goals and learned more about the idea of LGBTQ stress that we introduced in the prior chapter. In this chapter, we focused on how your specific experiences of LGBTQ-related stress—both in the past and more recent—might be related to your mental health today. Your work in this session will help to shape your experience with the rest of chapters and has the potential to help you become more aware of what is important to focus on as you move through this program.

This week, you also continued practicing a critical skill that we will continue in some of the future sessions: monitoring and recording your daily experiences to gain greater insight. Remember to think of this as what it is, "practice"—just like with sports, school, or hobbies, we only get better if we practice. If you get frustrated, that's OK—practice can be hard! Feel free to take a break. It can help to try out different times to work on the home practice exercises until you find the time that works for you. Remember, regular practice is more important than doing it "perfectly." Good luck and see you in the next chapter!

Home Practice: Monitoring LGBTQ-Related Stress

For this week's home practice exercise, please complete Worksheet 5.3: Monitoring LGBTQ-Related Stress—Understanding Emotion-Driven Behaviors to help you monitor and identify the *Before, During,* and *After* of your LGBTQ-related stress and emotions. Completing this worksheet will help you become aware of the types of LGBTQ-related stress that you face, maybe on a regular basis. The worksheet appears at the end of this chapter and is also available to download by searching for this book's title on the Oxford Academic platform at academic.oup.com. Figure 5.1 (on p. 66) shows an example of a completed worksheet (first column only).

Unfortunately, some of us "get used to" experiences of rejection or discomfort, which makes LGBTQ-related stress go unnoticed. By helping you identify LGBTQ-related stress, this exercise will help you understand possible causes for your negative mood.

As you can see on Worksheet 5.3, the columns are divided into:

- *Before*—What was the trigger?
- *During*—What was your emotional response (including thoughts, bodily feelings, and behaviors) to the trigger?
- *After*—What were the consequences of your emotional response?

For this chapter, we only want you to work on the first column (*Before*), which will require you to identify *triggering* situations that cause you to feel LGBTQ-related stress. For example, one trigger might be a stranger glaring at you or making a rude comment while you walk by holding hands with your partner, or altering your appearance, mannerisms, or activities to attempt to avoid anti-LGBTQ discrimination. Feel free to use any examples from this chapter that apply to you. Sometimes, individuals struggle to identify LGBTQ-related stressors. If this happens to you, feel free to broaden your monitoring for the first few days to include any triggers that cause stress, even those that are unrelated to LGBTQ stress.

In next week's chapter, we will look at your own examples to help you understand how these LGBTQ-related stressful situations may affect you and your emotions. You will also continue to monitor your weekly anxiety and depression symptoms.

Overall Depression Severity and Interference Scale (ODSIS)

Instructions: The following items ask about depression. For each item, indicate the number for the answer that best describes your experience over the past week.

—1. In the past week, how often have you felt depressed?

0 = **No depression** in the past week.

1 = **Infrequent depression**. Felt depressed a few times.

2 = **Occasional depression**. Felt depressed as much of the time as not.

3 = **Frequent depression**. Felt depressed most of the time.

4 = **Constant depression**. Felt depressed all of the time.

—2. In the past week, when you have felt depressed, how intense or severe was your depression?

0 = **Little or None**: Depression was absent or barely noticeable.

1 = **Mild**: Depression was at a low level.

2 = **Moderate**: Depression was intense at times.

3 = **Severe**: Depression was intense much of the time.

4 = **Extreme**: Depression was overwhelming.

—3. In the past week, how often did you have difficulty engaging in or being interested in activities you normally enjoy because of depression?

0 = **None**: I had no difficulty engaging in or being interested in activities that I normally enjoy because of depression.

1 = **Infrequent**: A few times I had difficulty engaging in or being interested in activities that I normally enjoy because of depression. My lifestyle was not affected.

2 = **Occasional**: I had some difficulty engaging in or being interested in activities that I normally enjoy because of depression. My lifestyle has only changed in minor ways.

3 = **Frequent**: I have considerable difficulty engaging in or being interested in activities that I normally enjoy because of depression. I have made significant changes in my lifestyle because of being unable to become interested in activities I used to enjoy.

4 = **All the Time**: I have been unable to participate in or be interested in activities that I normally enjoy because of depression. My lifestyle has been extensively affected and I no longer do things that I used to enjoy.

—4. In the past week, how much did your depression interfere with your ability to do the things you needed to do at work, at school, or at home?

0 = **None**: No interference at work/home/school from depression.

1 = **Mild**: My depression has caused some interference at work/home/school. Things are more difficult, but everything that needs to be done is still getting done.

2 = **Moderate**: My depression definitely interferes with tasks. Most things are still getting done, but few things are being done as well as in the past.

3 = **Severe**: My depression has really changed my ability to get things done. Some tasks are still being done, but many things are not. My performance has definitely suffered.

4 = **Extreme**: My depression has become incapacitating. I am unable to complete tasks and have had to leave school, have quit or been fired from my job, or have been unable to complete tasks at home and have faced consequences like bill collectors, eviction, etc.

—5. In the past week, how much has depression interfered with your social life and relationships?

0 = **None**: My depression doesn't affect my relationships.

1 = **Mild**: My depression slightly interferes with my relationships. Some of my friendships and other relationships have suffered, but, overall, my social life is still fulfilling.

2 = **Moderate**: I have experienced some interference with my social life, but I still have a few close relationships. I don't spend as much time with others as in the past, but I still socialize sometimes.

3 = **Severe**: My friendships and other relationships have suffered a lot because of depression. I do not enjoy social activities. I socialize very little.

4 = **Extreme**: My depression has completely disrupted my social activities. All of my relationships have suffered or ended. My family life is extremely strained.

Total Score: ____

Overall Anxiety Severity and Interference Scale (OASIS)

Instructions: The following items ask about anxiety and fear. For each item, indicate the number for the answer that best describes your experience over the past week.

—1. In the past week, how often have you felt anxious?

    0 = **No anxiety** in the past week.

    1 = **Infrequent anxiety.** Felt anxious a few times.

    2 = **Occasional anxiety.** Felt anxious as much of the time as not. It was hard to relax.

    3 = **Frequent anxiety.** Felt anxious most of the time. It was very difficult to relax.

    4 = **Constant anxiety.** Felt anxious all of the time and never really relaxed.

—2. In the past week, when you have felt anxious, how intense or severe was your anxiety?

    0 = **Little or None:** Anxiety was absent or barely noticeable.

    1 = **Mild:** Anxiety was at a low level. It was possible to relax when I tried. Physical symptoms were only slightly uncomfortable.

    2 = **Moderate:** Anxiety was distressing at times. It was hard to relax or concentrate, but I could do it if I tried. Physical symptoms were uncomfortable.

    3 = **Severe:** Anxiety was intense much of the time. It was very difficult to relax or focus on anything else. Physical symptoms were extremely uncomfortable.

    4 = **Extreme:** Anxiety was overwhelming. It was impossible to relax at all. Physical symptoms were unbearable.

—3. In the past week, how often did you avoid situations, places, objects, or activities because of anxiety or fear?

    0 = **None:** I do not avoid places, situations, activities, or things because of fear.

    1 = **Infrequent:** I avoid something once in a while, but will usually face the situation or confront the object. My lifestyle is not affected.

    2 = **Occasional:** I have some fear of certain situations, places, or objects, but it is still manageable. My lifestyle has only changed in minor ways. I always or almost always avoid the things I fear when I'm alone, but can handle them if someone comes with me.

    3 = **Frequent:** I have considerable fear and really try to avoid the things that frighten me. I have made significant changes in my lifestyle to avoid the object, situation, activity, or place.

    4 = **All the Time:** Avoiding objects, situations, activities, or places has taken over my life. My lifestyle has been extensively affected and I no longer do things that I used to enjoy.

—4. In the past week, how much did your anxiety interfere with your ability to do the things you needed to do at work, at school, or at home?

    0 = **None:** No interference at work/home/school from anxiety.

    1 = **Mild:** My anxiety has caused some interference at work/home/school. Things are more difficult, but everything that needs to be done is still getting done.

2 = **Moderate:** My anxiety definitely interferes with tasks. Most things are still getting done, but few things are being done as well as in the past.

3 = **Severe:** My anxiety has really changed my ability to get things done. Some tasks are still being done, but many things are not. My performance has definitely suffered.

4 = **Extreme:** My anxiety has become incapacitating. I am unable to complete tasks and have had to leave school, have quit or been fired from my job, or have been unable to complete tasks at home and have faced consequences like bill collectors, eviction, etc.

—5. In the past week, how much has anxiety interfered with your social life and relationships?

0 = **None:** My anxiety doesn't affect my relationships.

1 = **Mild:** My anxiety slightly interferes with my relationships. Some of my friendships and other relationships have suffered, but, overall, my social life is still fulfilling.

2 = **Moderate:** I have experienced some interference with my social life, but I still have a few close relationships. I don't spend as much time with others as in the past, but I still socialize sometimes.

3 = **Severe:** My friendships and other relationships have suffered a lot because of anxiety. I do not enjoy social activities. I socialize very little.

4 = **Extreme:** My anxiety has completely disrupted my social activities. All of my relationships have suffered or ended. My family life is extremely strained.

Total Score: ___

Progress Record

ODSIS

20	
18	
16	
14	
12	
10	
8	
6	
4	
2	
0	

Week 1 2 3 4 5 6 7 8 9 10 11 12 13 14 15 16 17 18 19 20 21 22 23 24 v

OASIS

20	
18	
16	
14	
12	
10	
8	
6	
4	
2	
0	

Week 1 2 3 4 5 6 7 8 9 10 11 12 13 14 15 16 17 18 19 20 21 22 23 24 v

Other Assessment

20	
18	
16	
14	
12	
10	
8	
6	
4	
2	
0	

Week 1 2 3 4 5 6 7 8 9 10 11 12 13 14 15 16 17 18 19 20 21 22 23 24 v

Worksheet 5.1: Examples of LGBTQ-Related Stress

Which of these examples apply to you now or in the past? Put a checkmark in the boxes to select all that apply.

Homophobia/Biphobia/ Transphobia	☐ Negative cultural/media depictions of LGBTQ people ☐ Not having the same legal rights as others ☐ Other people thinking that bisexual identities are not legitimate or real ☐ Being judged for being gender-nonconforming ☐ Other people thinking you are immoral or not religious because you are LGBTQ ☐ Feeling as if the spotlight is on you and that people can see right through you ☐ Unclear signals of potential rejection ☐ Fearing rejection ☐ Fearing hate crimes
Social Stress	☐ Social isolation ☐ Trouble finding a supportive community or friend group ☐ Feeling like an outcast ☐ Feeling like you are hiding, living a double life, or putting on a show ☐ Coming out, including planning when and whom to come out to ☐ Not being out causing strain on friendships ☐ Lack of LGBTQ role models ☐ Not trusting new people
Romantic Relationship Stress	☐ Avoiding romantic closeness ☐ Avoiding romantic feelings or statements like "I love you" ☐ Struggling to talk about HIV status ☐ Fearing getting HIV ☐ Pressure to hide your gender identity from romantic partners ☐ Pressure to lead a "straight" or "cis" life ☐ Pressure to be in a relationship ☐ Fleeting sexual encounters without lasting relationships ☐ Being bisexual or pansexual and feeling like others will think the gender identity of your current partner determines your sexual orientation ☐ Negotiating sexual agreements with partners
Family and Developmental Stress	☐ Early gender nonconformity ☐ Bullying ☐ Lack of parental acceptance ☐ Feelings of letting parents down ☐ Holidays highlighting non-accepting family members ☐ Family's misinformed theories about sexual orientation and/or gender identity ☐ Not having a sense of control

LGBTQ Community Stress	☐ Pressure to fit masculine or feminine norms ☐ Feeling like you are not being "queer enough" ☐ Rigid body standards and body image concerns ☐ Escaping difficult emotions or experiences through substances ☐ Easy validation and companionship through sex ☐ Rejection, invisibility, stereotypes, or discrimination within the LGBTQ community (e.g., racism, sexism, classism, ableism, ageism) ☐ Strong pressure to self-label ☐ Pressure to not label yourself as bisexual
Institutional Discrimination	Workplace Discrimination ☐ Getting passed up for a promotion ☐ Worrying about bringing your partner to work events ☐ Experiencing tokenism in the workplace (e.g., being a representative of all queer women) ☐ Feeling like you don't belong in your school/workplace because you are LGBTQ ☐ Not having gender-neutral bathrooms at work Healthcare Discrimination ☐ Challenges disclosing your sexual orientation to a health care provider ☐ Feeling judged or stereotyped by health care providers ☐ Reading questions on health care forms that exclude or invalidate your sexual orientation or gender identity ☐ Receiving mental health treatment from providers who view your sexual orientation as a pathology, phase, or form of confusion Educational Discrimination ☐ Being discriminated against in school admission decisions ☐ Not having openly LGBTQ teachers ☐ Never hearing about LGBTQ people in sex education ☐ Being prohibited or discouraged from publicly expressing affection or attending school dances ☐ Not learning about significant LGBTQ historical figures and events at school ☐ Being bullied for being LGBTQ ☐ Not having gender-neutral locker room options at school Religious Discrimination ☐ Being told your sexual orientation is a sin, a sign of evil or spiritual weakness, or worthy of punishment ☐ Hearing about or being forced to attend religious-based "conversion therapy" ☐ Being prohibited from holding an LGBTQ wedding ceremony within your place of worship ☐ Your religious/faith institution donating to anti-LGBTQ causes ☐ People of your sexual orientation/gender identity being prohibited from becoming religious leaders within your place of worship

Worksheet 5.2: LGBTQ-Related Stress Experiences and Emotions

First, consider the current situation you identified on page 58.

What was the immediate impact (right when the stressor occurred)?

What has been the ongoing impact (how does it still affect your emotions)?

Second, consider the past situation you identified on page 58.

What was the immediate impact (right when the stressor occurred)?

What has been the ongoing impact (how does it still affect your emotions)?

Worksheet 5.3: Monitoring LGBTQ-Related Stress–Understanding Emotion-Driven Behaviors

Before	During			After
Situations, Triggers	Thoughts	Behaviors	Bodily Feelings	Thoughts

Before	During			After
Situations, Triggers	Thoughts	Behaviors	Bodily Feelings	Thoughts
My partner didn't call when they said they would				
Friends didn't invite me out last night				
My Aunt used the wrong gender pronouns when referring to me during dinner				
Stranger sneered at me as I walked by holding my partner's hand				

Figure 5.1

Monitoring LGBTQ-Related Stress—Understanding Emotion-Driven Behaviors (First Column Completed as an Example)

| CHAPTER 6 | Module 3: Understanding and Tracking LGBTQ-Related Stress and Emotional Experiences |

Chapter 6 Overview

In this chapter, you will learn more about how emotions work and how they are relevant to you as an LGBTQ person. You will also learn how to understand and manage your emotions better. Just like the last chapter, you will also consider your experiences with LGBTQ-related stress to understand how it impacts your emotions.

Chapter 6 Outline

- Weekly Check-In
- Review Home Practice from Chapter 5
- What Are Emotions?
- The Three Parts of an Emotion
- How Are Emotions Relevant to LGBTQ People?
- What Is a Better Way of Coping With and Managing Your Emotions?
- Summary
- Home Practice: Observing and Tracking Your Emotional Responses

Take a minute to track your symptoms using the ODSIS and OASIS, located at the end of this chapter. You may also photocopy these forms or download multiple copies by searching for this book's title on the Oxford Academic platform at academic.oup.com. Do you notice any changes? What do you attribute these changes to?

Review Home Practice from Chapter 5

In the last chapter, you learned more about the many different kinds of LGBTQ-related stress. You started to figure out how it might be affecting your emotions and behaviors, particularly the ones that you want to change through this program.

You also started learning about the *Before*, *During*, and *After* of your LGBTQ-related stress experiences, and you specifically practiced identifying some *triggering* situations (*Before*) that lead to LGBTQ-related stress. On the lines below, write down the triggering situations you identified on Worksheet 5.3: Monitoring LGBTQ-Related Stress—Understanding Emotion-Driven Behaviors. Feel free to go back to the last chapter in order to review these situations—they'll be useful for the practice task this week. And remember, you're learning skills to cope wtih these situations and the stress they cause.

_____

_____

_____

_____

_____

_____

Last week you were also asked to monitor your weekly experiences of depression and anxiety by completing the ODSIS and OASIS. If you have not had the chance to complete these yet, please take a minute to do so.

- Are there any changes you're noticing related to depression and anxiety?
- Any changes you want to see happen?

In the coming weeks, we will help you identify the changes that you are making. We will also help you identify and overcome barriers to feeling better.

What Are Emotions?

Maybe you're like Juan, who feels anxious every time he goes to a party. He knows parties should be fun, but each time he goes he is consumed with fear about saying something stupid.

Or perhaps you're like Megan. She has spent years trying to build up the courage to ask someone out but can't seem to find the courage. Each time she gets close, she feels like she's going to panic and backs out.

Lastly, maybe you're in a situation like Kelly. They want to be more satisfied in their relationship, but no matter what they do, they can't seem to stop shutting down whenever their partner confronts them.

No matter your specific goals, it all starts with your emotions—what they are, how they work, and how to manage them.

You might be feeling scared about focusing on your emotions more. That's normal. Many people are hesitant to focus on difficult emotions. But it might help to remember something we discussed previously: Emotions themselves are not bad—even though they can feel pretty bad at times! Despite what you might think, it would actually be terrible if you never felt any negative emotions. That's because emotions tell us which events and situations we should pay attention to so that we can take action. Let's take a look at some common negative emotions to see why they are helpful and necessary:

Fear

Think of fear like you would think of your home smoke alarm, which goes off when there is potential danger in the house. You probably don't think of the smoke alarm in your house as a bad thing, right? You shouldn't think of fear in a negative way either—it's there to help you!

Imagine walking down the street and seeing a car quickly coming toward you. Your body instantly responds: Your heart starts racing, your eyes get bigger, and the muscles in your legs and arms tighten and prepare for action. Fear prompts you to jump out of the way of the car.

In this situation, fear is doing what it should—warning you about something dangerous so that you do something to save your life.

Sadness

We usually get sad after a loss or setback of some sort—a break-up, the death of someone we care about, or unmet expectations. We often feel sadness when there is a big difference between our actual life and how we want our life to be.

Sadness tells us to pull back and re-evaluate a loss or setback. For example, feeling sad after a break-up lets you know that the relationship was important to you. Sadness might prompt you to take time to process your experience of the relationship and its ending, which may help you be more successful in your next relationship. Sadness also lets others know that we need support and draws them to us.

Anxiety

Anxiety is an emotion that helps us prepare for the future. It tells us that important or dangerous situations might occur. When we feel anxious, it encourages us to focus our attention on whatever is causing the anxiety so that we can attempt to prevent a bad outcome.

Feeling anxious before a presentation at work focuses your attention on the task so that you can properly prepare for it. What do you think would happen if you felt no anxiety before a big presentation? You probably wouldn't feel the motivation to prepare for it and would not do as well as you could.

It's possible you might think: "OK, I get it. I understand how fear can save me from an oncoming car or someone coming to attack me. But what about the fear I have when I go on a first date? That seems ridiculous and out of place. Or what about the anxiety I feel when I'm at a party? How is that helping me? It's overwhelming me and ruining my life."

These are all valid points. Some emotions might not make sense at first. Sometimes emotions appear to be completely random, or way more intense than they need to be given the situation we are in. Sometimes anxiety "misfires" in situations where there is not an actual threat. Some of this is due to a person's history, and some of us are just wired to have more anxiety than others. Why does this happen? The short answer lies in how we respond to the different parts of our emotions *when they occur*.

The Three Parts of an Emotion

To understand your emotions better, let's first look at the three parts of an emotion.

1. Bodily Feelings (How You Feel in Your Body)

Every emotion you have is linked with some kind of physical feeling. Your body goes through physical changes when you feel an emotion. For example, when you feel afraid, you might have a faster heartbeat, tenser muscles, and quicker breathing. Let's apply this idea to your experiences.

What physical feelings come with feeling *excited*?

_____

_____

What about *anger*?

_____

_____

How about *embarrassment*?

_____

_____

2. Thoughts (What You Think)

The way you think about a situation really changes how you feel about it. For example, if you go up to someone to ask them on a date while thinking thoughts like "They will probably reject me" or "They are out of my league, and I don't stand a chance," then you will likely feel sad, afraid, or ashamed. If you feel sad or ashamed, you're more likely to have negative thoughts about yourself or the situation. Let's apply this idea to your experiences.

What thoughts did you have the last time you felt *anxious*?

_____

_____

What about the last time you felt *angry*?

_____

_____

How about the last time you felt *guilty*?

_____

_____

3. Behaviors (What You Do)

Whenever you feel an emotion, it comes with the urge to act. Earlier, we talked about how some urges to act can be helpful (such as jumping out of the way when a car is coming at you). But sometimes our behaviors are not so helpful. For example, someone who is sad may isolate themselves from others and watch television all day. Or someone who is anxious about going to a party might leave as soon as they feel anxious.

These kinds of behaviors are called *emotion-driven behaviors*. They are the behaviors we engage in, usually automatically, when we feel intense emotions. And often these automatic behaviors are what keep us trapped in our unhappiness. Think about what you do or feel like doing when you experience the following emotions:

What do you do (or feel like doing) when you're *sad*?

_____

_____

What about when you're *angry*?

_____

_____

What about when you're *ashamed* or *embarrassed*?

_____

_____

Putting This All Together

These three parts—feelings, thoughts, and behaviors—happen every time we experience an emotion. Some of these parts might be easier for you to identify than the others. It's important to pay attention to all three and how they interact with one another to understand our emotions better.

To practice identifying these three parts of emotional experiences, let's look at an example from Ari:

Ari feels anxious most of the time—with his friends, at work, and even when he's at home by himself. To understand his constant anxiety better, he broke his anxiety down into the three parts we just talked about. Take a look at Box 6.1 on page 89, which is Ari's completed Worksheet 6.1: Three-Component Model of Emotions. We will talk later about how Ari can use this breakdown to handle his anxiety better. For now, Ari is just trying to *understand* his anxiety.

Now, it's your turn. Using Worksheet 6.1 at the end of this chapter, think of a negative emotion you experienced this past week. Try to break it down into your feelings, thoughts, and behaviors. You may also download a copy of this worksheet by searching for this book's title on the Oxford Academic platform at academic.oup.com.

How Are Emotions Relevant to LGBTQ People?

Research shows that LGBTQ people are more likely to have a hard time with emotions than straight, cisgender people. That's because many LGBTQ individuals have pushed away their feelings and interests since childhood in order to feel that they are staying safe and fit in. Take Justin for example:

As a kid, Justin had different interests than other boys his age. He enjoyed singing, drama, and dolls. Because of these interests, Justin was teased endlessly by other boys in his class. As a result, Justin learned to hide his interests and instead pretended to be interested in sports, cars, and action movies. Although Justin had no interest in these things, he pretended to like them when he was at school to keep from getting teased.

Because LGBTQ people are constantly reminded that they are different, they can experience uncomfortable emotions over and over again, multiple times a day. Because these emotions can be unpleasant, it makes total sense for someone's first reaction to be to push away or avoid them. However, this can sometimes get us into trouble. As all people do, we repeat things that make us feel better and avoid things that make us feel bad. Just like Justin, many LGBTQ people have gotten used to pushing away emotions to avoid feeling bad. This can sometimes lead LGBTQ folks to push away *all* feelings and to perceive emotions as dangerous.

Here is another example:

When Jìngyi was a child, she was bullied by other girls for playing sports, wearing athletic clothing every day, and hanging mostly with boys. Jìngyi learned at a young age to not show the other girls how badly they were hurting her feelings. So, she began to ignore and push away the negative emotions she felt when she got teased.

We repeat things that make us feel better and avoid things that make us feel bad. Just like Justin and Jìngyi, many LGBTQ people form a pattern of repeatedly pushing away emotions to avoid feeling bad. People push away emotions in many different ways, including thinking about negative things over and over; avoiding other people, avoiding speaking up, or avoiding intimacy; and using alcohol, drugs, or sex. This often leads to a vicious cycle: The more a person engages in these types of emotion-driven behaviors, the more normal these responses become. This can prevent new learning from happening.

Because of this, many LGBTQ people may not have fully experienced anxiety or sadness since a young age or at all. They may not have learned that these emotions are safe and potentially helpful.

While avoiding emotions may have been helpful in some early situations, these strategies often have negative consequences when used over and over. For example:

As an adult, Justin often feels like he isn't close to anyone. He wants to be close with others but is not sure how to do it. His early way of connecting with others was to hide his true self. As a result, he now has a deeply held belief that people will dislike him once they get to know who he really is. So, he avoids intimacy with others. He ends relationships before they get too serious and often uses sarcasm to prevent conversations with his friends from getting too intimate.

Jìngyì is now 30 and still manages her emotions the same way she did when she was a child. When she experiences an uncomfortable emotion, she ignores and pushes it away. However, as she has gotten older, the emotions have gotten more intense and harder to ignore. As a result, Jìngyì uses alcohol to help her dull the emotions. She has several drinks per day and often gets drunk by herself at home.

Can you see how your early experiences with LGBTQ-related stress might shape you as an LGBTQ person? Can you think of any examples of LGBTQ-related stress from your past that shaped how you manage your emotions today?

Keep these examples in mind because we'll work with them later in this chapter.

What Is a Better Way of Coping With and Managing Your Emotions?

It's much easier to cope with emotions when we know when, where, and why they happen. To do this, you will need to look more closely at your emotional experiences, monitor what is happening in those experiences, and take note of what happened before and after you experienced an emotion.

To help you with this, think of your emotional experiences as having three parts:

1. *Before* (Remember this from the last chapter?)—Your emotion didn't come out of nowhere. Sometimes an event or trigger happened a lot earlier and sometimes it happened right before your emotion.

For example, a stranger might sneer at you in the morning when you walk by them with your partner, and this could change the way you approach an afternoon phone call at work. You might have a harder time concentrating or worry about doing something wrong on the call.

2. *During*—This refers to the thoughts, physical feelings, and behaviors that make up an emotional response. These are the three parts of emotions we just learned about. Together, these three things form your response to the event or trigger.

3. *After*—This refers to what you experience as a result of your responses (in other words, the consequences) and can be both short and long term. Consequences affect how you behave when you experience the same emotion again. For example, say you're at a party (*Before*) and you start to feel social anxiety, so you leave the party (*During*), causing your anxiety to go away quickly (*After*). In the future, you will likely leave a party early again when you feel anxious (because it led to short-term relief of your social anxiety).

These three parts (*Before*, *During*, and *After*) give us some insight into our experiences and why we feel the way we do. Let's look at one of Justin's examples.

Justin felt depressed and sad when his friends did not invite him out with them last Saturday night.

1. *Before*—Not getting invited to go out with his friends was the trigger.

2. *During*—Justin responded to this trigger by *thinking* that no one liked him and that he was unlovable. As a result, he *felt* inferior, lonely, and sad. This resulted in *behaviors* like giving his friends the silent treatment and avoiding them.

3. *After*—Because of this experience, Justin started declining future social invitations. As a result, his friends stopped inviting him out as much because he usually said no. Now, to fill his weekends, Justin usually stays in to work extra hours from home.

Do you see how the before, during, and after are all connected to each other in Justin's example?

During this week's home practice, you'll try breaking down some of your own emotional experiences with LGBTQ-related stress just like we did for Justin here.

Summary

In this chapter, you learned about how your emotions, even the negative ones, can be helpful tools to help you navigate life. As you know now, the thoughts, feelings, and behaviors that emotional responses come with can sometimes form patterns over time that are hard to break and aren't helpful in the long run. LGBTQ people in particular can develop emotional responses that don't work for them due to life-long experiences of LGBTQ-related stress. However, you can develop an understanding of how to better monitor emotional experiences in your own life, monitoring the *Before* and *After* of an experience as well as the parts of an emotional response while you're feeling it (*During*). This isn't an easy task, but it does get easier with practice and experience over time.

Home Practice: Observing and Tracking Your Emotional Responses

Building off the last chapter's home practice, let's practice examining some of your own emotional experiences with LGBTQ-related stress from the past week.

Using Worksheet 6.2: Monitoring LGBTQ-Related Stress, located at the end of this chapter, write down some of your experiences, and see if you can identify the *Before*, *During*, and *After* in each of your examples. You may also download a copy of this worksheet by searching for this book's title on the Oxford Academic platform at academic.oup.com. Table 6.1 (on pp. 91) show you how to do this. Remember, in addition to tracking your triggers (*Before*), this week you will also be paying attention to your response thoughts, physical feelings, and behaviors (*During*) and both the short- and long-term consequences (*After*).

Though it may be awkward at first, actively tracking your emotional experiences can be very helpful.

This week, practice this kind of tracking each time you experience a strong emotion (or at least once a day). Tracking these experiences throughout the week will hopefully get you to notice patterns in your emotional experiences. With this awareness, you can start the process of changing your responses!

Think of this as "practice"— just like with sports, school, or hobbies, we only get better if we practice. If you get frustrated, that's OK—practice can be hard! Feel free to take a break. It can help to try out different times to work on the exercises until you find the time that works for you.

Remember: Regular practice is more important than doing it "perfectly." Good luck, and we're looking forward to sharing some strategies for handling strong emotions in the next chapter!

Overall Depression Severity and Interference Scale (ODSIS)

Instructions: The following items ask about depression. For each item, indicate the number for the answer that best describes your experience over the past week.

—1. In the past week, how often have you felt depressed?

0 = **No depression** in the past week.

1 = **Infrequent depression**. Felt depressed a few times.

2 = **Occasional depression**. Felt depressed as much of the time as not.

3 = **Frequent depression**. Felt depressed most of the time.

4 = **Constant depression**. Felt depressed all of the time.

—2. In the past week, when you have felt depressed, how intense or severe was your depression?

0 = **Little or None**: Depression was absent or barely noticeable.

1 = **Mild**: Depression was at a low level.

2 = **Moderate**: Depression was intense at times.

3 = **Severe**: Depression was intense much of the time.

4 = **Extreme**: Depression was overwhelming.

—3. In the past week, how often did you have difficulty engaging in or being interested in activities you normally enjoy because of depression?

0 = **None**: I had no difficulty engaging in or being interested in activities that I normally enjoy because of depression.

1 = **Infrequent**: A few times I had difficulty engaging in or being interested in activities that I normally enjoy because of depression. My lifestyle was not affected.

2 = **Occasional**: I had some difficulty engaging in or being interested in activities that I normally enjoy because of depression. My lifestyle has only changed in minor ways.

3 = **Frequent**: I have considerable difficulty engaging in or being interested in activities that I normally enjoy because of depression. I have made significant changes in my lifestyle because of being unable to become interested in activities I used to enjoy.

4 = **All the Time**: I have been unable to participate in or be interested in activities that I normally enjoy because of depression. My lifestyle has been extensively affected and I no longer do things that I used to enjoy.

—4. In the past week, how much did your depression interfere with your ability to do the things you needed to do at work, at school, or at home?

0 = **None**: No interference at work/home/school from depression.

1 = **Mild**: My depression has caused some interference at work/home/school. Things are more difficult, but everything that needs to be done is still getting done.

2 = **Moderate**: My depression definitely interferes with tasks. Most things are still getting done, but few things are being done as well as in the past.

3 = **Severe**: My depression has really changed my ability to get things done. Some tasks are still being done, but many things are not. My performance has definitely suffered.

4 = **Extreme**: My depression has become incapacitating. I am unable to complete tasks and have had to leave school, have quit or been fired from my job, or have been unable to complete tasks at home and have faced consequences like bill collectors, eviction, etc.

—5. In the past week, how much has depression interfered with your social life and relationships?

0 = **None**: My depression doesn't affect my relationships.

1 = **Mild**: My depression slightly interferes with my relationships. Some of my friendships and other relationships have suffered, but, overall, my social life is still fulfilling.

2 = **Moderate**: I have experienced some interference with my social life, but I still have a few close relationships. I don't spend as much time with others as in the past, but I still socialize sometimes.

3 = **Severe**: My friendships and other relationships have suffered a lot because of depression. I do not enjoy social activities. I socialize very little.

4 = **Extreme**: My depression has completely disrupted my social activities. All of my relationships have suffered or ended. My family life is extremely strained.

Total Score: ____

Overall Anxiety Severity and Interference Scale (OASIS)

Instructions: The following items ask about anxiety and fear. For each item, indicate the number for the answer that best describes your experience over the past week.

—1. In the past week, how often have you felt anxious?

    0 = **No anxiety** in the past week.

    1 = **Infrequent anxiety.** Felt anxious a few times.

    2 = **Occasional anxiety.** Felt anxious as much of the time as not. It was hard to relax.

    3 = **Frequent anxiety.** Felt anxious most of the time. It was very difficult to relax.

    4 = **Constant anxiety.** Felt anxious all of the time and never really relaxed.

—2. In the past week, when you have felt anxious, how intense or severe was your anxiety?

    0 = **Little or None:** Anxiety was absent or barely noticeable.

    1 = **Mild:** Anxiety was at a low level. It was possible to relax when I tried. Physical symptoms were only slightly uncomfortable.

    2 = **Moderate:** Anxiety was distressing at times. It was hard to relax or concentrate, but I could do it if I tried. Physical symptoms were uncomfortable.

    3 = **Severe:** Anxiety was intense much of the time. It was very difficult to relax or focus on anything else. Physical symptoms were extremely uncomfortable.

    4 = **Extreme:** Anxiety was overwhelming. It was impossible to relax at all. Physical symptoms were unbearable.

—3. In the past week, how often did you avoid situations, places, objects, or activities because of anxiety or fear?

    0 = **None:** I do not avoid places, situations, activities, or things because of fear.

    1 = **Infrequent:** I avoid something once in a while, but will usually face the situation or confront the object. My lifestyle is not affected.

    2 = **Occasional:** I have some fear of certain situations, places, or objects, but it is still manageable. My lifestyle has only changed in minor ways. I always or almost always avoid the things I fear when I'm alone, but can handle them if someone comes with me.

    3 = **Frequent:** I have considerable fear and really try to avoid the things that frighten me. I have made significant changes in my lifestyle to avoid the object, situation, activity, or place.

    4 = **All the Time:** Avoiding objects, situations, activities, or places has taken over my life. My lifestyle has been extensively affected and I no longer do things that I used to enjoy.

—4. In the past week, how much did your anxiety interfere with your ability to do the things you needed to do at work, at school, or at home?

    0 = **None:** No interference at work/home/school from anxiety.

    1 = **Mild:** My anxiety has caused some interference at work/home/school. Things are more difficult, but everything that needs to be done is still getting done.

2 = **Moderate:** My anxiety definitely interferes with tasks. Most things are still getting done, but few things are being done as well as in the past.

3 = **Severe:** My anxiety has really changed my ability to get things done. Some tasks are still being done, but many things are not. My performance has definitely suffered.

4 = **Extreme:** My anxiety has become incapacitating. I am unable to complete tasks and have had to leave school, have quit or been fired from my job, or have been unable to complete tasks at home and have faced consequences like bill collectors, eviction, etc.

—5. In the past week, how much has anxiety interfered with your social life and relationships?

0 = **None:** My anxiety doesn't affect my relationships.

1 = **Mild:** My anxiety slightly interferes with my relationships. Some of my friendships and other relationships have suffered, but, overall, my social life is still fulfilling.

2 = **Moderate:** I have experienced some interference with my social life, but I still have a few close relationships. I don't spend as much time with others as in the past, but I still socialize sometimes.

3 = **Severe:** My friendships and other relationships have suffered a lot because of anxiety. I do not enjoy social activities. I socialize very little.

4 = **Extreme:** My anxiety has completely disrupted my social activities. All of my relationships have suffered or ended. My family life is extremely strained.

Total Score: ___

Progress Record

ODSIS

```
20 ─────────────────────────────────────────
18 ─────────────────────────────────────────
16 ─────────────────────────────────────────
14 ─────────────────────────────────────────
12 ─────────────────────────────────────────
10 ─────────────────────────────────────────
 8 ─────────────────────────────────────────
 6 ─────────────────────────────────────────
 4 ─────────────────────────────────────────
 2 ─────────────────────────────────────────
 0 ─────────────────────────────────────────
```

| Week 1 | 2 | 3 | 4 | 5 | 6 | 7 | 8 | 9 | 10 | 11 | 12 | 13 | 14 | 15 | 16 | 17 | 18 | 19 | 20 | 21 | 22 | 23 | 24 | v |

OASIS

```
20 ─────────────────────────────────────────
18 ─────────────────────────────────────────
16 ─────────────────────────────────────────
14 ─────────────────────────────────────────
12 ─────────────────────────────────────────
10 ─────────────────────────────────────────
 8 ─────────────────────────────────────────
 6 ─────────────────────────────────────────
 4 ─────────────────────────────────────────
 2 ─────────────────────────────────────────
 0 ─────────────────────────────────────────
```

| Week 1 | 2 | 3 | 4 | 5 | 6 | 7 | 8 | 9 | 10 | 11 | 12 | 13 | 14 | 15 | 16 | 17 | 18 | 19 | 20 | 21 | 22 | 23 | 24 | v |

Other Assessment

```
20 ─────────────────────────────────────────
18 ─────────────────────────────────────────
16 ─────────────────────────────────────────
14 ─────────────────────────────────────────
12 ─────────────────────────────────────────
10 ─────────────────────────────────────────
 8 ─────────────────────────────────────────
 6 ─────────────────────────────────────────
 4 ─────────────────────────────────────────
 2 ─────────────────────────────────────────
 0 ─────────────────────────────────────────
```

| Week 1 | 2 | 3 | 4 | 5 | 6 | 7 | 8 | 9 | 10 | 11 | 12 | 13 | 14 | 15 | 16 | 17 | 18 | 19 | 20 | 21 | 22 | 23 | 24 | v |

Worksheet 6.1: Three-Component Model of Emotions

1. Cognitive (What I Think): These are the thoughts often triggered by or linked with feeling states.
2. Behavioral (What I Do): These are actions a person engages in or has the urge to engage in as a response to the feeling state. Often, someone will respond to a feeling without thinking about it. This is because it seems like our bodies just "know" the best way to deal with these situations. As noted above, these are behaviors.
3. Bodily Feelings (How I Feel in My Body): These are the bodily feelings attached to emotional states.

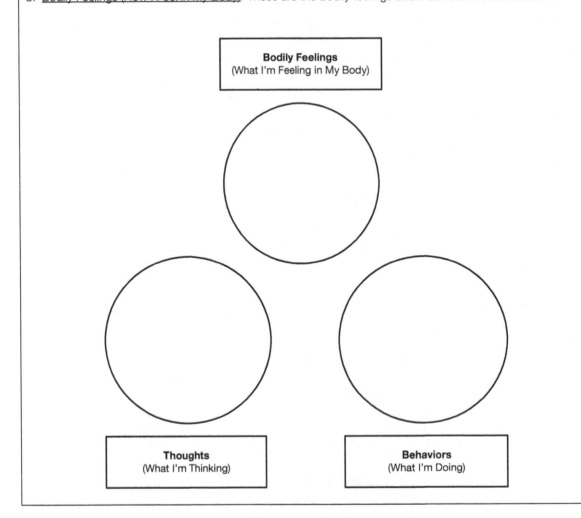

Box 6.1. Ari's Completed Worksheet 6.1: Three-Component Model of Emotions

1. <u>Cognitive (What I Think)</u>: These are the thoughts often triggered by or linked with feeling states.
2. <u>Behavioral (What I Do)</u>: These are actions a person engages in or has the urge to engage in as a response to the feeling state. Often, someone will respond to a feeling without thinking about it. This is because it seems like our bodies just "know" the best way to deal with these situations. As noted above, these are learned behaviors.
3. <u>Bodily Feelings (How I Feel in My Body)</u>: These are the bodily feelings attached to emotional states.

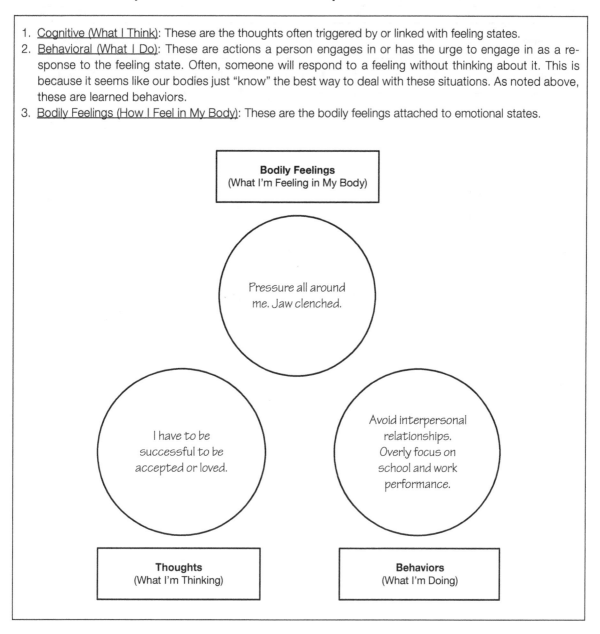

Worksheet 6.2: Monitoring LGBTQ-Related Stress

Before	During			After
Situations, Triggers	Thoughts	Behaviors	Bodily Feelings	Thoughts

Table 6.1. Justin's Completed Worksheet 6.2: Monitoring LGBTQ-Related Stress

Before	During			After
Situations, Triggers	Thoughts	Behaviors	Bodily Feelings	Thoughts
My partner didn't call when they said they would.	What's wrong with me?	Isolated myself in my room. Didn't go out with my friends while I waited for my partner to call.	Warm in my face, hot all over.	Couldn't sleep well while thinking about my deficiencies over and over.
Friends didn't invite me out last night.	No one likes me; I'm not lovable; I will never have close friends.	Avoided social situations. Tried to focus on things I am good at, like work.	Sinking feeling in my stomach. Numb.	Turned down social invitations in order to go over work I already finished.
My Aunt used the wrong gender pronouns when referring to me during dinner.	I'm too complicated; my gender is a burden to others.	Consumed more alcohol than I'd planned to.	Heaviness in my entire body.	Made multiple expensive "impulse purchases" online later that night.
Stranger sneered at me as I walked by holding my partner's hand.	People will never accept us. I shouldn't even try.	Made sure my feelings didn't show on my face. Let go of my partner's hand.	Tingling in my fingers and arms, then a knot in my stomach.	Denied being upset when my partner asked and decided not to join them at dinner with their family that night.

Module 4: Increasing Mindful Awareness of LGBTQ-Related Stress Reactions

Chapter 7 Overview

This program is designed, in general, to help you manage negative emotions in more helpful ways. This chapter will increase your ability to experience emotions in the moment, with fuller acceptance and less judgment. To accomplish this, the chapter will introduce you to the concept of *nonjudgmental emotion awareness*, or mindfulness, and provide opportunities to practice it within your daily life. This present-focused awareness is a first step towards finding better ways to cope with emotions. Over time, this skill can help you to not only face your emotions, but also to accept them, allow them to pass, and learn from them.

Chapter 7 Outline

- Weekly Check-In
- Review Home Practice from Chapter 6
- LGBTQ-Related Stress and Emotional Coping
- Importance of Emotion Awareness
- Nonjudgmental Emotion Awareness
- Practicing Nonjudgmental Emotion Awareness
- Summary
- Home Practice 1: Nonjudgmental, Present-Focused Emotion Awareness
- Home Practice 2: Anchoring in the Present
- Home Practice 3: Nonjudgmental, Present-Focused Emotion Awareness by Recreating an Emotional State

Weekly Check-In

Take a minute to track your symptoms using the ODSIS and OASIS, located at the end of this chapter. You may also photocopy these forms or download multiple copies by searching for this book's title on the Oxford Academic platform at academic.oup.com. Do you notice any changes? What do you attribute these changes to?

Review Home Practice from Chapter 6

In the last chapter, you learned about emotions and the ways that feelings, thoughts, and behaviors affect each other. You also learned that past, negative LGBTQ-related experiences can affect how you react to situations today. Reflect on what you learned by considering the following questions:

1. What did you learn from tracking the *Before*, *During*, and *After* of your emotional experiences last week when you completed Worksheet 6.2: Monitoring LGBTQ-Related Stress? Take a moment, reflect on your experience, and write down any patterns you noticed.

   _____

   _____

   _____

2. Were there any parts of the tracking task that were more challenging for you? Write down ideas of how you can continue noticing the *Before*, *During*, and *After* of your intense emotional experiences moving forward.

   _____

   _____

   _____

LGBTQ-Related Stress and Emotional Coping

Everyday stress can lead to uncomfortable emotions. LGBTQ people, in particular, might experience strong uncomfortable emotions because their everyday stress builds on top of their LGBTQ-related stress to make them feel more stress overall and to feel this stress more strongly. How we learn to cope with stress—both general stress and LGBTQ-related stress—can determine how strongly we feel our uncomfortable emotions. Some LGBTQ people may have learned coping strategies for stress that feel good in the short term because they make the unpleasant emotions less intense. However, these strategies can become unhelpful in the long term and actually lead to more uncomfortable emotions because they prevent us from facing our emotions, feeling them, and learning from them.

Remember Justin and Jìngyì from the previous chapter? They each developed ways of coping with LGBTQ-related stress as children that were not very helpful ways of coping with stress as adults. Here are some more examples:

- Sonia is not out to her friends at work. She constantly worries about accidentally saying she is gay. She is quiet at work and never talks about her personal life, choosing instead to work really hard at her desk all the time.
- Andreyei gets clammy and feels like running away whenever they go to a bar to try and meet people. But, after three or four drinks, they find that this feeling goes away, and they are able to talk to anyone. So now, Andreyei always has a few drinks at home before going out.

Sonia and Andreyei have figured out ways to help them navigate stressful situations in their everyday lives. Both of these coping strategies have one thing in common—they allow Sonia and Andreyei to cope by escaping uncomfortable emotions that make them feel vulnerable. But both of them are avoiding the uncomfortable emotions, rather than engaging with them.

Why might these coping strategies be unhelpful for Sonia and Andreyei in the long run?

_____

_____

Think of three ways in which *you* avoid feeling uncomfortable or vulnerable.

1. _____

2. _____

3. _____

Write about one or two coping strategies that you use that seem helpful now but might not be the most helpful in the long term. Write down why they may not be helpful:

1. _____

_____

_____

2. _____

_____

_____

Importance of Emotion Awareness

Because avoidance can make us feel better and reduce negative emotions in the short term, it can become our go-to strategy for coping with negative emotions. However, avoidance prevents us from facing emotions, feeling them, and learning from them. In fact, continually avoiding our emotions can actually make those emotions bigger and more uncomfortable in the long term. This is because as long as we avoid emotions, we can never get used to them and learn about them and our relationship to them, which paradoxically makes them easier to tolerate.

As we discussed in the previous chapter, anxiety and depression can lead people to view any sort of emotion—even positive emotions, like joy—as threatening and unpleasant. People who are anxious or depressed often interpret their emotions as having disastrous results, rather than as feelings that come and go. However, it's very important to remember that while these interpretations of emotions are not very helpful, for a lot of LGBTQ individuals, these reactions have developed from previous negative experiences with these emotions.

For LGBTQ folks, early experiences of rejection, shame, and isolation can lead to us having a hard time identifying and expressing how we're feeling. This is because we were often told that our emotions are bad and we therefore developed coping strategies to try to not feel uncomfortable emotions.

How can we break this cycle of avoiding emotions? One way is to allow ourselves to experience emotions as they are happening, rather than suppressing or avoiding them. And in order to do that, we need to focus on what is happening in the present.

Consider Levi:

Until middle school, Levi had a large group of friends and mostly got along with everyone in his classes. Then Levi's friends started dating each other and other classmates. Levi knew that unlike his closest friends, he had romantic feelings for boys, not girls. But Levi also knew that if he came out, his classmates might make fun of him or stop talking to him. So, he said nothing and hid his feelings towards boys. Whenever someone asked him about who he liked, he changed the subject.

Now, Levi is in his 20s and out to nearly everyone in his life. He is dating, but every time a date goes badly, he is devastated. More and more, Levi finds himself avoiding dating, choosing instead to meet people only for anonymous hookups, often while drunk or high. He has learned to avoid his uncomfortable emotions by trying to not feel anything.

Perhaps you don't identify with Levi. Maybe you feel like you feel your feelings *all the time* and that your feelings are confusing, overwhelming, or seem to just "happen automatically" without your control. Remember, when we experience emotions, they are often a mix of feelings, physical sensations, and *thoughts* about these sensations. This mix of reactions together can feel overwhelming.

Important to understanding your emotional reaction to stress is to consider that your emotional reaction can be broken down into two parts—a primary emotion and a secondary reaction.

Primary emotional reactions arise first. For example:

Vincent has been job-searching for a while and feels anxious about an upcoming interview. Anxiety is his primary emotion. But when he is anxious, he immediately starts beating himself up for feeling that way.

A moderate amount of anxiety before a big event can be helpful because it can provide the push to prepare for what's coming. But the way that Vincent starts blaming himself for feeling anxious is unhelpful. His self-blame is not an emotion, but rather a judgment of his emotion. This is his secondary reaction to his primary emotion of anxiety. Unfortunately, this secondary judgment only serves to increase his anxiety more.

Secondary reactions, like judging our emotions, or feeling shame or guilt about them, can lead us to view emotions as something threatening and unwanted. Instead, we could see emotions as our body's clever way of signaling to us what is going on in our world *right now*.

Let's think about Levi again. When he is rejected, his primary emotion is sadness. This sadness is accompanied by a secondary reaction — judgment about himself, being rejected, and being sad. For instance, when he feels sad after being rejected, he thinks, "I'm going to feel this way forever" and "I shouldn't feel this way."

These secondary judgments are not emotions. Instead, they are a *response* to the sad feelings that Levi experiences when things don't work out with a partner. Levi reacts to these emotions and judgments the way he learned to when he was younger, by burying them and avoiding situations where he might be rejected.

Think back to a time when *you* were feeling sad or depressed. You may find that in addition to feeling sadness or depression you had thoughts like, "I will always feel this way" or "Why can't I be happy?" or "Why can't I deal with it?" These secondary thoughts are responses to your sadness.

Sometimes, we can even have negative reactions to *positive emotions*. Take Bridget, for example:

Bridget has been hooking up with a new partner who she really likes. But whenever her partner says something nice and loving, Bridget immediately responds with a critical remark. Bridget might be thinking, "If I let this go on, something bad might happen. I could get hurt."

Growing up in an environment without models of happy, healthy queer relationships, Bridget internalized the idea that happy queer relationships are impossible. To Bridget, it could be dangerous to feel happy or loved in a queer relationship because it might lead to hurt feelings or sadness. Rather than accept her positive, happy feelings as an indication that things are going well in her relationship, she shuts them down and tries to suppress them. Her response has the unintentional impact of making her and her partner more stressed.

Often, secondary reactions to emotions are not based on what is happening in front of us. They are based on what happened before, or what we worry might happen in the future. Sometimes when we experience an unpleasant emotion, we focus on what happened when we last felt that way or what might happen if we feel it again in the future. So, we lose sight of the fact that *none of that is currently happening*.

Think of Vincent and his upcoming job interview: in the moment, it is neither true that Vincent is messing up his interview, nor true that he will never get a job. What is happening is that Vincent has an interview for a job, and the outcome of the interview is unknown.

Try to identify a recent stressful situation which caused *you* to feel strong emotions. What was your primary emotion?

_____

_____

Can you identify a secondary reaction to that primary emotion?

_____

_____

Nonjudgmental Emotion Awareness

You might be thinking, "OK, how does this help my anxiety or depression? And what exactly does being aware of my emotions even involve?"

Being aware of judgments that you might have towards your emotions can help you understand how judgments affect your behaviors. This is where the practice of nonjudgmental emotion awareness comes in.

Nonjudgmental emotion awareness means purposefully focusing your attention on the present moment. This involves observing the thoughts, physical feelings, and behaviors that happen in response to your emotions. But it does not involve judging the fact that you are having these emotions, or judging the emotions themselves. You are practicing being neutral about the fact that you are having emotions. By observing your experience without judgment, you can accept your emotions as they are without trying to change them.

"Alright, so how does this *help* me?"

Being in touch with your emotions as they are happening and practicing *feeling* them, instead of avoiding them, can stop you from going back to old, unhelpful coping strategies. This can be a first step towards finding new, helpful strategies. Over time, you might even begin to learn things from your emotions, such as identifying your values or things you want to change in your life. You may also find that your negative emotions pass more quickly than you expect.

Note that we're not changing your reactions yet. Think of nonjudgmental emotion awareness as an emergency brake for when you feel your emotions carrying you away. Right now, we're just practicing being in better touch with emotions that feel overwhelming. In later chapters, we will discuss how you can use this present-focused awareness to be in charge of your emotions, rather than letting them determine how you react to situations.

Practicing Nonjudgmental Emotion Awareness

Activity 1: Mindfulness Meditation

Becoming aware of your emotions requires practice. Your emotions may have been getting the best of you for a long time now. It will take time to change that pattern.

It might feel scary to focus so intently on emotions—especially if you're used to avoiding them. But remember, engaging with our emotions helps us to manage them better in the long term.

To help you get started, let's try a quick mindfulness exercise. If you are working with a therapist, they may read this exercise aloud to you during session. The audio file for this exercise (called "Activity 1: Mindfulness Meditation") can also be downloaded by searching for this book's title on the Oxford Academic platform at academic.oup.com, so that you can listen to the meditation on your own.

When you're ready, settle into your chair—try sitting comfortably upright, setting both feet on the ground, resting your arms and hands in a comfortable position. As you settle in, begin to notice the rise and fall of your breath. Simply notice your breath as it is. There is no need to count, change, or do anything different with your breathing. Just let it be and observe it as it currently is.

Begin to scan your body, noticing the sensations in your muscles, your heartbeat, and your breath. You might also notice the sensations of your feet touching the ground, your body in your chair, or your arms resting on your lap. Just observe these physical sensations, without judgment or evaluation. As you sit and become present to your current physical state, begin to notice what is happening in your mind. Notice what feelings you're currently experiencing. If you notice a specific feeling, try describing it without evaluation. If you notice sadness, you can imagine the word "sad." If you notice anxiety, you can imagine the word "anxious." If you notice happiness, imagine the word "happy." This lets you notice and describe your current state of being, without judging it.

As you sit and tune in to your thoughts, feelings, and physical sensations, remember that there is no need to change, judge, or avoid your current experiences. Right now, all you are asked to do is notice and let it be. Continuing to be present to your current state of being, notice what thoughts your mind is producing at this time. Imagine that you are watching your thoughts being produced as though they're a movie you are watching. In this way, you can stop yourself from getting "hooked" into the thoughts, and instead just watch them play out as an objective observer. If, as you strive to be present and self-aware in the here and now, you find yourself getting carried away by thoughts about the past or future, that's OK. Try using your breath as an anchor to bring yourself back into the present moment. Notice the physical sensation of the breath you are taking right now. In this way, you can always use your breath to anchor you to the present moment.

You might also notice judgments or evaluations that you have in response to your emotions. You might have the thought, "This emotion is bad" or "I shouldn't feel this way." You could also think, "I like this feeling and I don't want it to go away." If you notice any of these reactions, gently bring yourself back to the role of an objective observer. If you notice you are feeling sad, you can think the word "sad" or if you notice you are anxious, you can think of the word "anxious." Know that there is no right or wrong way to feel. All you are asked to do right now is to notice and describe your current feelings.

Bringing your full attention back to your breath, notice a few more breaths, then when you're ready, you can bring yourself back into the room.

Reflect on this exercise. What emotions came up for you? Did you notice any secondary judgments of those emotions?

_____

_____

_____

Notice how thoughts and judgments of thoughts arise all the time.

Activity 2: Mood Induction

In stressful situations, we can get carried away and return to old unhelpful patterns because they may be the only way we know how to cope. Practicing nonjudgmental awareness can help us pause and stop our automatic coping strategies from taking over. This can help us realize that the distressing emotion will pass and that it doesn't need to guide our behaviors. This can be the first step towards developing more helpful coping strategies.

Let's practice nonjudgmental emotion awareness.

Think about an LGBTQ-related stressful experience that you had recently and can remember vividly. Feel free to revisit Worksheet 6.2: Monitoring LGBTQ-Related Stress if that is helpful.

Write down your experience in a few words:

_____

_____

Now you are going to try bringing yourself back to that particular moment to practice being aware of what emotions you felt in that moment. You will also practice observing what judgments you had about those emotions at the time.

Remember, being present-focused and self-aware sometimes means tolerating difficult feelings. Try to practice observing your emotions without judgment and without trying to change the emotions you feel. If you are working with a therapist, they may read this exercise aloud to you during session. The audio file for this exercise (called "Activity 2: Mood Induction") can also be downloaded by searching for this book's title on the Oxford Academic platform at academic.oup.com, so that you can listen to the meditation on your own.

Sitting comfortably in your chair, begin to recall this experience in as much detail as possible. Remember where you were; who was there; and what you saw, heard, or felt in that moment. Try thinking about the situation as though it were happening to you all over again.

As you take yourself back to that situation, begin to notice the physical sensations that you are experiencing. What do you notice in your body? Notice your breath, heartbeat, muscles, and any other physical sensation you experience. Remember, there is no need to change how you feel. Simply notice your experiences, without judgment or evaluation.

Now begin to notice what feelings you are experiencing. You may notice different types of emotions. Try just naming those emotions that you detect. You might notice feelings of sadness, nervousness, worry, happiness. There is no right or wrong way to feel. Just notice your feelings, letting them be. Notice the thoughts that you are experiencing, having put yourself back in this situation. Our minds are factories of thoughts—try simply watching those thoughts being produced by your mind, as an independent and objective observer.

If you find yourself becoming hooked into ruminating about the past or worrying about the future, try bringing your attention back to your breath as a way of becoming present to the here and now. Try asking yourself, "What am I thinking about <u>right now</u>? "How am I feeling <u>right now</u>? What am I doing <u>right now</u>?

Notice a few more breaths, and when you are ready, bring yourself back to the room.

What did you notice during the exercise? About your feelings? About your thoughts? About your behaviors?

_____

_____

_____

Maybe you found yourself getting "carried away" by remembering emotions from that day. Or perhaps you noticed judging yourself for getting carried away by thoughts. Maybe you had the thought that you weren't doing this right. Don't worry! There is no right or wrong way to practice present-focused awareness.

This is a skill you might be learning for the first time. As with anything you are learning for the first time, don't expect yourself to be able to do it "perfectly" from the start. The first time you rode a bike, did you just jump on and pedal off into the distance? Or did you fall, maybe several times, before you were able to ride the bike well?

When you are observing your experience in this way, you might find your thoughts carrying you away a hundred times, and that's OK! You can "get back on track" by refocusing your attention every time you notice your thoughts carrying you away, until eventually it gets easier. The very fact that you notice yourself getting carried away by your thoughts means you *are* successfully observing your experience!

Just like any other skill, being focused on the present takes practice before it becomes something you do easily.

An Example of Using Mindfulness in a Stressful Situation

Think back to Worksheet 6.1: Three-Component Model of Emotions from the last chapter—including thoughts, behaviors, and bodily feelings.

Remember Vincent and his job interview from earlier in this chapter? Figure 7.1 separates Vincent's experience according to the Model of Emotions. His thoughts of the worst-case scenario happening—messing up the job interview—are increasing the anxiety he already has about the interview. This leads Vincent to avoid preparing for the interview instead

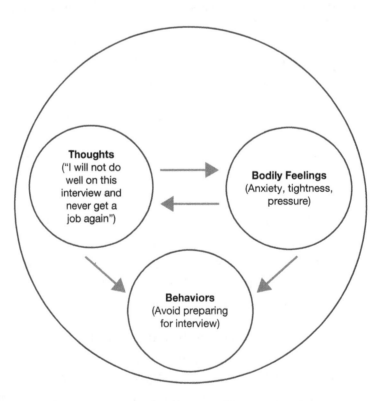

Figure 7.1

Example of Thoughts, Behaviors, and Bodily Feelings in a Stressful Situation of approaching his anxiety and looking up things about the company that could help him succeed at the interview.

Practicing nonjudgmental awareness could help Vincent to pause, notice his thoughts and feelings, and allow his anxiety to pass. This mindful approach could help him take an observer's perspective and help him identify how his thoughts, emotions, and behaviors are affecting each other in the moment.

When you're in the middle of your emotional experience, sometimes it can be hard to distance yourself from it. You can try a useful "cue" to help you practice bringing your attention back to the present if you find yourself getting carried away by your emotions.

The cue is a mini-version of the exercise that you just practiced and is called the "three-point check." If you find yourself getting overwhelmed by your emotions, you can take a deep breath and ask yourself three questions:

1. Ask yourself, **"What am I *feeling* right now?"**
   Maybe you find yourself feeling anxious. Imagine the word "anxious." Try spelling out "anxious" in your mind.
2. Ask yourself, **"What am I *thinking* about right now?"**
   Maybe thoughts like, "I can't cope with this situation" or "I'll never get anything done" are increasing your anxiety.
3. Ask yourself, **"What am I *doing* right now?"**
   This final question can turn your attention away from the thoughts and feelings that are overwhelming and bring you back to focusing on what's going on right now.

You can use the three-point check at any time as a cue to help you focus on what's happening in the present. Just ask yourself those three questions.

Summary

This chapter focused on allowing yourself to experience emotions in the present moment, with full acceptance and without judgment. As you have now learned, it is common for LGBTQ people to suppress negative emotions as a result of LGBTQ stress. In this chapter, you practiced present-focused nonjudgmental awareness to cope with stress. Observing emotional experiences mindfully is not easy. Practicing what you've learned in this chapter will be helpful for future chapters, especially in allowing you to better describe your experiences.

Home Practice 1: Nonjudgmental, Present-Focused Emotion Awareness

Set aside some time every day this week to practice nonjudgmental emotion awareness. It could just be five minutes per day to start off. Right now, you are being asked to practice with time you set aside, but over time this will become more automatic.

In the beginning, it may seem awkward or hard to practice being aware of your emotions using this approach. Use the practice exercises (the audio files, which you can download and listen to on your own) and the three-point check at least once per day to help you get started. Over time, you may find it easier and easier to stop judging your emotions, which is the first step towards managing them better!

Think of this as practice. Just like with sports, school, or hobbies, we only get better at things through frequent practice. If you find yourself feeling frustrated, that's OK—practice can be hard sometimes. Feel free to take a break, or try completing these home practices at different times each day to figure out what works best for you. Doing the practice *regularly* is more important than doing it *perfectly*. Good luck!

Use Worksheet 7.1: Nonjudgmental, Present-Focused Emotion Awareness at the end of this chapter to practice being aware of your emotions in the present moment, in a nonjudgmental way, and see how they affect your thoughts and behaviors. You may also download a copy of this worksheet by searching for this book's title on the Oxford Academic platform at academic.oup.com. Every morning and evening this week, take a few minutes to practice checking in with yourself and noticing your thoughts, feelings, and reactions or behaviors happening *at that moment*. Try using the three-point check.

As an example, Andreyei's use of the three-point check is shown in the first row of Worksheet 7.1. They ask themself:

- *What am I feeling right now?*
- *What am I thinking about right now?*
- *What am I doing right now?*

As you complete the worksheet, also notice the judgments that arise along with your thoughts and emotions. Write down how much you were able to accept emotions in the moment and not judge them. You may find fewer and fewer judgments arising as you continue to practice.

Home Practice 2: Anchoring in the Present

For the second practice this week, you will anchor yourself in the present at least three times by noticing at least one thing going on around you for at least 60 seconds and recording this on Worksheet 7.2: Anchoring in the Present, located at the end of this chapter. You may also download a copy of this worksheet by searching for this book's title on the Oxford Academic platform at academic.oup.com. This anchor can be a sound you hear, something you see, or something you can physically feel (like a chair, a computer keyboard, or a dish sponge). You can also use your breath to help bring your attention to the present moment. Whatever anchor you choose, let this become a reminder to shift your attention to the present moment. Remember that the goal of this exercise is not to think about the meaning of what you notice, nor is it to try to understand your reaction to it. The purpose of this exercise is simply to practice paying attention to what is going on around you at that moment.

Home Practice 3: Nonjudgmental, Present-Focused Emotion Awareness by Recreating an Emotional State

For the third home practice this week, you will practice nonjudgmental emotion awareness by recreating an emotional state and noticing the thoughts, physical feelings, and behaviors that come up. To help you get started, you can select a reminder of LGBTQ-related stress from your own life that has strong memories or personal meaning associated with it. Reminders can be photographs, letters, video clips, old emails, or even a song that has personal meaning and brings up strong emotions for you. As you listen or watch, notice your reaction and use Worksheet 7.3: Mood Induction Recording to record your experience. As you practice this exercise, try to note your reactions to these reminders: What was your first emotional response? How strongly did you feel these initial emotions? What was your reaction to this initial emotional response—what thoughts, sensations, or feelings did you experience? Try completing this exercise for at least five minutes on one day per week.

The worksheet is located at the end of this chapter; you may also download a copy by searching for this book's title on the Oxford Academic platform at academic.oup.com.

The first row of Worksheet 7.3 has been filled in for you, as an example. Try completing this worksheet at least two times this week to notice what thoughts and feelings come up for you when you are experiencing a strong emotion.

Overall Depression Severity and Interference Scale (ODSIS)

Instructions: The following items ask about depression. For each item, indicate the number for the answer that best describes your experience over the past week.

—1. In the past week, how often have you felt depressed?

    0 = **No depression** in the past week.

    1 = **Infrequent depression**. Felt depressed a few times.

    2 = **Occasional depression**. Felt depressed as much of the time as not.

    3 = **Frequent depression**. Felt depressed most of the time.

    4 = **Constant depression**. Felt depressed all of the time.

—2. In the past week, when you have felt depressed, how intense or severe was your depression?

    0 = **Little or None**: Depression was absent or barely noticeable.

    1 = **Mild**: Depression was at a low level.

    2 = **Moderate**: Depression was intense at times.

    3 = **Severe**: Depression was intense much of the time.

    4 = **Extreme**: Depression was overwhelming.

—3. In the past week, how often did you have difficulty engaging in or being interested in activities you normally enjoy because of depression?

    0 = **None**: I had no difficulty engaging in or being interested in activities that I normally enjoy because of depression.

    1 = **Infrequent**: A few times I had difficulty engaging in or being interested in activities that I normally enjoy because of depression. My lifestyle was not affected.

    2 = **Occasional**: I had some difficulty engaging in or being interested in activities that I normally enjoy because of depression. My lifestyle has only changed in minor ways.

    3 = **Frequent**: I have considerable difficulty engaging in or being interested in activities that I normally enjoy because of depression. I have made significant changes in my lifestyle because of being unable to become interested in activities I used to enjoy.

    4 = **All the Time**: I have been unable to participate in or be interested in activities that I normally enjoy because of depression. My lifestyle has been extensively affected and I no longer do things that I used to enjoy.

—4. In the past week, how much did your depression interfere with your ability to do the things you needed to do at work, at school, or at home?

    0 = **None**: No interference at work/home/school from depression.

    1 = **Mild**: My depression has caused some interference at work/home/school. Things are more difficult, but everything that needs to be done is still getting done.

    2 = **Moderate**: My depression definitely interferes with tasks. Most things are still getting done, but few things are being done as well as in the past.

    3 = **Severe**: My depression has really changed my ability to get things done. Some tasks are still being done, but many things are not. My performance has definitely suffered.

4 = **Extreme**: My depression has become incapacitating. I am unable to complete tasks and have had to leave school, have quit or been fired from my job, or have been unable to complete tasks at home and have faced consequences like bill collectors, eviction, etc.

—5. In the past week, how much has depression interfered with your social life and relationships?

0 = **None**: My depression doesn't affect my relationships.

1 = **Mild**: My depression slightly interferes with my relationships. Some of my friendships and other relationships have suffered, but, overall, my social life is still fulfilling.

2 = **Moderate**: I have experienced some interference with my social life, but I still have a few close relationships. I don't spend as much time with others as in the past, but I still socialize sometimes.

3 = **Severe**: My friendships and other relationships have suffered a lot because of depression. I do not enjoy social activities. I socialize very little.

4 = **Extreme**: My depression has completely disrupted my social activities. All of my relationships have suffered or ended. My family life is extremely strained.

Total Score: ___

Overall Anxiety Severity and Interference Scale (OASIS)

Instructions: The following items ask about anxiety and fear. For each item, indicate the number for the answer that best describes your experience over the past week.

—1. In the past week, how often have you felt anxious?

0 = **No anxiety** in the past week.

1 = **Infrequent anxiety.** Felt anxious a few times.

2 = **Occasional anxiety.** Felt anxious as much of the time as not. It was hard to relax.

3 = **Frequent anxiety.** Felt anxious most of the time. It was very difficult to relax.

4 = **Constant anxiety.** Felt anxious all of the time and never really relaxed.

—2. In the past week, when you have felt anxious, how intense or severe was your anxiety?

0 = **Little or None:** Anxiety was absent or barely noticeable.

1 = **Mild:** Anxiety was at a low level. It was possible to relax when I tried. Physical symptoms were only slightly uncomfortable.

2 = **Moderate:** Anxiety was distressing at times. It was hard to relax or concentrate, but I could do it if I tried. Physical symptoms were uncomfortable.

3 = **Severe:** Anxiety was intense much of the time. It was very difficult to relax or focus on anything else. Physical symptoms were extremely uncomfortable.

4 = **Extreme:** Anxiety was overwhelming. It was impossible to relax at all. Physical symptoms were unbearable.

—3. In the past week, how often did you avoid situations, places, objects, or activities because of anxiety or fear?

0 = **None:** I do not avoid places, situations, activities, or things because of fear.

1 = **Infrequent:** I avoid something once in a while, but will usually face the situation or confront the object. My lifestyle is not affected.

2 = **Occasional:** I have some fear of certain situations, places, or objects, but it is still manageable. My lifestyle has only changed in minor ways. I always or almost always avoid the things I fear when I'm alone, but can handle them if someone comes with me.

3 = **Frequent:** I have considerable fear and really try to avoid the things that frighten me. I have made significant changes in my lifestyle to avoid the object, situation, activity, or place.

4 = **All the Time:** Avoiding objects, situations, activities, or places has taken over my life. My lifestyle has been extensively affected and I no longer do things that I used to enjoy.

—4. In the past week, how much did your anxiety interfere with your ability to do the things you needed to do at work, at school, or at home?

0 = **None:** No interference at work/home/school from anxiety.

1 = **Mild:** My anxiety has caused some interference at work/home/school. Things are more difficult, but everything that needs to be done is still getting done.

2 = **Moderate:** My anxiety definitely interferes with tasks. Most things are still getting done, but few things are being done as well as in the past.

3 = **Severe:** My anxiety has really changed my ability to get things done. Some tasks are still being done, but many things are not. My performance has definitely suffered.

4 = **Extreme:** My anxiety has become incapacitating. I am unable to complete tasks and have had to leave school, have quit or been fired from my job, or have been unable to complete tasks at home and have faced consequences like bill collectors, eviction, etc.

—5. In the past week, how much has anxiety interfered with your social life and relationships?

0 = **None:** My anxiety doesn't affect my relationships.

1 = **Mild:** My anxiety slightly interferes with my relationships. Some of my friendships and other relationships have suffered, but, overall, my social life is still fulfilling.

2 = **Moderate:** I have experienced some interference with my social life, but I still have a few close relationships. I don't spend as much time with others as in the past, but I still socialize sometimes.

3 = **Severe:** My friendships and other relationships have suffered a lot because of anxiety. I do not enjoy social activities. I socialize very little.

4 = **Extreme:** My anxiety has completely disrupted my social activities. All of my relationships have suffered or ended. My family life is extremely strained.

Total Score: ___

Progress Record

ODSIS

```
20 ────────────────────────────────────────────
18 ────────────────────────────────────────────
16 ────────────────────────────────────────────
14 ────────────────────────────────────────────
12 ────────────────────────────────────────────
10 ────────────────────────────────────────────
 8 ────────────────────────────────────────────
 6 ────────────────────────────────────────────
 4 ────────────────────────────────────────────
 2 ────────────────────────────────────────────
 0 ────────────────────────────────────────────
```

| Week 1 2 3 4 5 6 7 8 9 10 11 12 13 14 15 16 17 18 19 20 21 22 23 24 v |

OASIS

```
20 ────────────────────────────────────────────
18 ────────────────────────────────────────────
16 ────────────────────────────────────────────
14 ────────────────────────────────────────────
12 ────────────────────────────────────────────
10 ────────────────────────────────────────────
 8 ────────────────────────────────────────────
 6 ────────────────────────────────────────────
 4 ────────────────────────────────────────────
 2 ────────────────────────────────────────────
 0 ────────────────────────────────────────────
```

| Week 1 2 3 4 5 6 7 8 9 10 11 12 13 14 15 16 17 18 19 20 21 22 23 24 v |

Other Assessment

```
20 ────────────────────────────────────────────
18 ────────────────────────────────────────────
16 ────────────────────────────────────────────
14 ────────────────────────────────────────────
12 ────────────────────────────────────────────
10 ────────────────────────────────────────────
 8 ────────────────────────────────────────────
 6 ────────────────────────────────────────────
 4 ────────────────────────────────────────────
 2 ────────────────────────────────────────────
 0 ────────────────────────────────────────────
```

| Week 1 2 3 4 5 6 7 8 9 10 11 12 13 14 15 16 17 18 19 20 21 22 23 24 v |

Worksheet 7.1: Nonjudgmental, Present-Focused Emotion Awareness

	What did you notice?			How Effective Were You at Not Judging Your Experience?
	Thoughts	**Behaviors**	**Bodily Feelings**	**0 --------------------- 10** (not at all) (extremely)
Andreyei's example	I can't talk to anyone; I'm never going to find a partner	Getting a drink	Anxiety; feeling sweaty and clammy; urge to drink	1
Sun				
Mon				
Tues				
Wed				
Thurs				
Fri				
Sat				

Worksheet 7.2: Anchoring in the Present

	What Did You Notice?	How Effective Were You at Anchoring Yourself in the Present? 0 -------------------- 10 (not at all) (extremely)
	the sound of rain dropping on the pavement	6
Sun		
Mon		
Tues		
Wed		
Thurs		
Fri		
Sat		

Worksheet 7.3: Mood Induction Recording

Rate the intensity of your emotional experience using the 0- to 10-point scale below:

Reminder (e.g., photograph, letter, song)	Initial Emotional Response (Describe emotions you experienced)	Intensity of Emotional Response (Rate how strongly you felt these emotions) 0------------ 10 (not at all) (extremely)	Reaction to Emotional Response		
			Describe Thoughts	Describe Behaviors (e.g., fidgeting, pacing, sighing)	Describe Bodily Feelings
Coming-out letter that I wrote to my parents	Happiness mixed with sadness and nostalgia	7	I was so emotional back then. I also understand why I needed to tell them.	sighing, cringing	felt jittery, tightness in chest, heart sank

CHAPTER 8   Module 5: Increasing Cognitive Flexibility

Chapter 8 Overview

In this chapter you will explore the impact of LGBTQ-related stress on your thoughts, including negative opinions you may have about yourself, others, and your future. You will also learn to identify your stressful ways of thinking.

Chapter 8 Outline

- Weekly Check-In
- Review Home Practice from Chapter 7
- Activity: Identify Your Automatic Thoughts
- The Nature and Function of Automatic Thoughts
- LGBTQ-Related Stress and Automatic Thoughts
- Core Beliefs
- Common Thinking Traps
- Flexible Thinking Can Overcome Stressful Automatic Thoughts
- Flexible Thinking and LGBTQ-Related Stress
- Some Important Notes
- Summary
- Home Practice: Identifying, Testing, and Changing Your Automatic Thoughts

Weekly Check-In

Take a minute to track your symptoms using the ODSIS and OASIS, located at the end of this chapter. You may also photocopy these forms or download multiple copies by searching for this book's title on the Oxford Academic platform at academic.oup.com. Do you notice any changes? What do you attribute these changes to?

Review Home Practice from Chapter 7

How did it go practicing nonjudgmental emotion awareness? Were you able to practice nonjudgmental emotion awareness every day? List any obstacles that came up as you practiced nonjudgmental emotional awareness:

_____

_____

Is there any particular time that works better for you to practice in the coming weeks? Before bedtime? While walking? First thing in the morning? Write down your responses:

_____

_____

Did you notice any changes in your experience of emotion awareness over the week?

_____

_____

Activity: Identify Your Automatic Thoughts

Take a look at the mock text message exchange in Figure 8.1. Imagine you are the sender, texting first with a group of friends and then later with one member of your friend group, Dakota.

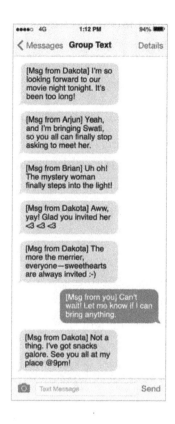
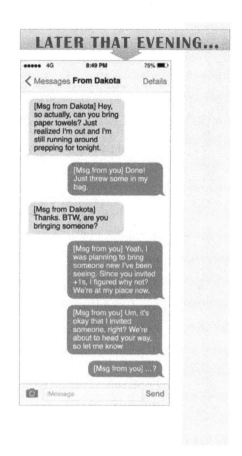

Figure 8.1

Ambiguous Experience Example

Write down your first thoughts about what happened at the end of the text exchange. Going forward, we'll refer to these first thoughts as your "automatic interpretations" or "automatic thoughts."

_____

_____

In any given situation or interaction, we can focus on many different aspects of what has taken place. The meaning that our mind gives to those aspects then predicts what we think might happen in that event in the moment or in the future. This process often happens without us being aware of it. How we interpret an event is influenced by several things:

1. how we are feeling in that moment;
2. clues we take from the current context; and
3. our past experiences.

What do you think influenced your automatic interpretation of the text exchange above?

_____

_____

For instance, perhaps you focused on a specific line within the text thread. Maybe you focused on Dakota's participation in the group text versus Dakota's exchange with you. Or maybe you remembered a similar situation when you were treated differently because of your sexual orientation or gender identity.

Maybe your mood right now influenced your initial thought. If you feel down and depressed today, you might have thought Dakota was uncomfortable with you bringing the person you've been seeing. If you feel happy and upbeat today, you might have thought she is probably rushing to get ready for the party and truly feels "the more the merrier."

How did your current mood affect your automatic thoughts about the text exchange?

_____

_____

The Nature and Function of Automatic Thoughts

Our automatic thoughts are the first thoughts we have about new situations. These thoughts help us filter out unimportant information so we can respond quickly. Often, it is useful to focus on only a few key pieces of information (e.g., the facial expressions of your partner during a conversation) while ignoring other information (e.g., the sounds of cars honking during the conversation).

Over time, we develop a particular way of interpreting situations. This can be really helpful to us. For example, because we've been to grocery stores before, we know how they work. We _automatically_ know what to do when we enter a grocery store. We don't need to consciously think about each step.

Now, returning to the text conversation with Dakota, try to think flexibly. Try to come up with at least three _new_ interpretations of the picture.

If your first interpretation was negative (for example, Dakota is rejecting you or Dakota is anti-LGBTQ) try to come up with some positive ones (for example, Dakota is busy preparing to host the gathering and will be excited to meet your guest), and vice versa. Write your alternative interpretations down here. The goal is to practice *flexible* thinking—even if you have to get creative in your new interpretations:

1. _____

2. _____

3. _____

How do these new thoughts make you feel? Write down those feelings:

1. _____

2. _____

3. _____

LGBTQ-Related Stress and Automatic Thoughts

On the one hand, automatic thinking can be helpful in some situations. It's probably helped you to interpret a situation automatically—that's why you've continued to do it! On the other hand, sometimes our automatic thinking can be unhelpful, which can lead to negative consequences like depression, anxiety, or substance use.

Research shows that because LGBTQ people often have negative experiences, like being rejected, bullied, or having to hide our true selves, we are more likely than heterosexual or cisgender people to have negative thinking styles, which can cause depression or anxiety.

We learn about ourselves, our world, and our future possible selves in a society that often holds negative views of LGBTQ individuals. Parental and peer support protects LGBTQ people from experiencing distress. However, this support isn't guaranteed, and stigmatizing messages have an impact.

Take Jenner:

As a little boy, Jenner's favorite color was pink and he played with dolls, whereas his brothers were athletic and played football. His parents were never proud of Jenner the way they were of his brothers. They only acknowledged him when he got good grades. In college, Jenner came out as gay and began embracing the more feminine aspects of his gender expression. His parents disowned him. Although he was deeply hurt, he threw himself into studying even more, which helped boost his self-esteem.

Now 28 years old, Jenner's life is not going as planned. He thought he would be making a lot of money and married with a family by now. However, he's single and makes only enough money to get by. He is sure no man would want to date "a loser" like him. As a result, he feels really down and depressed and has avoided making friends or dating.

Some research has actually found that Jenner's way of coping—basing his self-worth on getting good grades and other achievements—is particularly common among some LGBTQ people. Specifically, because of the demands of LGBTQ-related stress, like early concealment and expectations of rejection, LGBTQ people might base their self-worth on achievements like academics, work, appearance, and competition, possibly because other forms of self-esteem, like family approval, are not always available to LGBTQ people.

Let's consider Annalisa:

Annalisa grew up in a conservative, religious community that openly disapproved of same-sex relationships. At 12 years old, she realized she was attracted to other girls but hid it from everyone she knew so she wouldn't be rejected. She kept her conversations surface-level, never allowing anyone to get too close.

Now at age 24, Annalisa has been openly bisexual for several years. However, she is always anxious and self-conscious in social and romantic situations. She doesn't feel comfortable making decisions or sharing what she thinks. She always goes along with what everyone else wants and often questions whether she said the right thing. She tends to bottle things up until she blows up, which others don't like.

For both Jenner and Annalisa, early experiences shaped their automatic thoughts. They tend to really notice negative things, especially things that could mean they will be rejected (like someone averting their eyes). Jenner's avoidance of dating is driven by his *thought*, "I have nothing to offer." As a result, he is always on guard, looking for signs that he is disliked. Annalisa's fear of sharing her feelings is driven by her *thought* that "if they knew the true me, I would be rejected." She looks for signs that others don't like her.

The way both Jenner and Annalisa were treated when they were growing up has caused them to have negative automatic thoughts about themselves and how others perceive and relate to them.

Write down how you think your experiences growing up shaped what kind of information you pay attention to in different situations:

_____

_____

_____

People often hide their LGBTQ identities as teenagers and even as adults. This period of hiding may make LGBTQ individuals sensitive to the threat of being "found out" or rejected. It may also make LGBTQ people try really hard to fit in so that they can avoid rejection. Some LGBTQ people learn to fit in by pretending to be "straight" or more masculine/ feminine than they really are.

Experiencing LGBTQ-related stress while growing up can change the way LGBTQ people think. For example, being rejected for being LGBTQ can lead us to expect future rejection or to believe we are unlovable across our relationships.

Some LGBTQ people say that threats of rejection or not fitting in can also come from the LGBTQ community itself. For example, some LGBTQ people describe the community as "obsessed" with good looks and youth, leading folks to fear not being accepted because of the way they look or their age. Others describe rigid rules in the LGBTQ community about how masculine or feminine a person should look.

Take Jasper:

Jasper is a queer man who is a few pounds heavier than he'd like to be. He feels pretty insecure about his body, especially because his gay friends always say mean things about other men's bodies that are similar to his. Recently, Jasper started using apps to meet dates, and a guy he was interested in told him he wasn't into "chubby guys." Jasper can't stop thinking he'll be single forever. He feels depressed and thinks that his dreams of having a husband and family won't happen for him and that life seems pointless now.

What Is a Core Belief?

All of the thoughts described above can guide our expectations for how others will treat us as well as guide our thoughts about ourselves and our futures. Over time, these messages can become *core beliefs*—that is, beliefs that are formed because of past experiences, which get easily triggered by situations that seem similar.

Remember the text exchange shown in Figure 8.1?

You might have found it difficult to come up with a new interpretation to challenge your automatic interpretation. Or, you may have come up with other interpretations but had a hard time believing them. You may also notice when you do this in your real life that it's really hard to consider other perspectives when you are feeling a strong negative emotion.

To help you better understand what a core belief is, think of a stressful situation you've been in. It can be a situation like the text exchange or something else. Write it down in a few words here:

_____

We'll refer back to this situation throughout the chapter. Take a look at Worksheet 8.1: Downward Arrow Technique, located at the end of this chapter. You may also download a copy of this worksheet by searching for this book's title on the Oxford Academic platform at academic.oup.com. You'll see that you can identify your core beliefs by asking yourself a series of questions about your initial thoughts in a stressful situation. You can identify your initial thought, also called an automatic thought, by asking yourself: "What does this stressful situation mean about me?" After you have a sense of your automatic thought, you can identify your core belief by asking yourself: "If this were true, what would it mean about me?" "Why does this matter to me?" "What would happen if this were true?" "What would happen next?"

By asking yourself these questions, you can identify your own core beliefs.

To see an example of how to identify your core beliefs in response to a stressful situation, take a look at Figure 8.2: Downward Arrow Technique—LGBTQ-Related Stress Example, located at the end of this chapter just after Worksheet 8.1. In this figure, you'll see the example of Andal, their stressful situation ("Some friends went out last night without inviting me"), and their responses.

Common core beliefs among LGBTQ people include:

1. *Expectations of rejection* (e.g., "No one will ever love me;" "If I say what I want, I'll be rejected;" "If people know who I really am, they won't like me")
2. *Internalized transphobia or homophobia* (e.g., "Being trans makes me bad;" "I and other gay men are inferior, lower status, or diseased")
3. *Contingent self-worth* (e.g., "If I fail at something, I'm unlovable;" "I have to win to have value as a person").

Do any of these common core beliefs fit with your experience? If so, write down how:

_____

_____

If so, where do you think you may have learned these lessons?

_____

_____

Andal's core belief, "I'm unlovable," made them feel ashamed, lonely, self-conscious, inadequate, and embarrassed. Their physical feelings were shortness of breath, tight chest, fast heartbeat, and muscle tension in their neck and back. How do your core beliefs make you feel?

_____

_____

Recognizing our core beliefs is usually painful: It can be difficult, but powerful, to face the negative things we believe about ourselves.

Take some time before proceeding if you need to. The good news is that in this chapter you are soon going to learn ways to combat your core beliefs so they don't have as much power over your emotions and behaviors.

Why Are Your Core Beliefs Unhelpful to You?

Andal realized that their core belief of being unlovable made them feel even worse. This led them to isolate from others, which made them feel lonelier. Then, to deal with the pain, they drank excessively, which goes against their goals of reducing their alcohol intake and handling stress without substances.

Often our negative automatic thoughts are a watered-down version of our core belief. For example, Andal's core belief, "I'm unlovable," eventually came out in how they automatically interpreted the experience of not being invited out with their friends. They didn't initially think, "Oh, the reason they didn't invite me out is because I'm unlovable." Instead, they automatically thought a less intense version of that core belief: "I knew they never liked me." Like Andal, when you look closer, you can usually see how your core belief influences negative thoughts about yourself and interactions with others.

Starting to Change Your Core Beliefs

After you've thought of some alternatives to your core beliefs, look for evidence supporting the new core belief each day. This can be things that happen to you or things that you do well. For example:

Andal began to practice remembering their new core thought, "I'm lovable." They noticed that a friend complimented them and that a fellow trans person within their community invited them to a birthday party.

You will still experience and notice negative events, but try to *also* look for positive things that could support your new core belief. It may help to write two or three things down each day.

Common Thinking Traps

To start to develop more flexible ways of thinking instead of so frequently jumping to negative interpretations, as is common in depression and anxiety, it can be helpful to analyze the components of a stressful situation and your reactions to them. Worksheet 8.2: Identifying and Evaluating Automatic Thoughts can help you do that. This worksheet is located at the end of this chapter and also available for download by searching for this book's title on the Oxford Academic platform at academic.oup.com. Using this worksheet, first write down the details of the stressful situation in the left-hand column. Then, in the second column, write down your automatic thoughts or interpretations. In the third column, write down the emotions you felt in the situation. You can use the completed example shown in Figure 8.3: Identifying and Evaluating Automatic Thoughts—LGBTQ-Related Stress Examples (also located at the end of this chapter) as a guide.

After you've jotted down the situation and your automatic thoughts and emotions in that situation, you can categorize your automatic thoughts into your typical "thinking traps." Let's take a look at two common types of thinking traps.

Jumping to Conclusions

Jumping to conclusions is when we believe the chance of something bad happening is higher than the actual chance of it happening. For example, Elka is *100% certain* that if she tried to talk to a potential romantic partner, her anxiety would be so overwhelming that she would not be able to say one word. In reality, the chance of something bad happening is probably quite low.

Besides not being able to talk, what else could happen in Elka's situation that's not quite so bad (and maybe even quite positive)?

_____

_____

_____

Thinking the Worst

Thinking the worst is when we overestimate how badly something is going to go while underestimating our ability to handle it—in other words, expecting the *worst* possible outcome. Zephyr is *100% certain* that if they were to tell their boss that they were non-binary, their boss would refuse to use their pronouns, make jokes about them in front of coworkers, and spread rumors about them that block them from future promotions. In reality, a variety of positive and/or negative reactions are possible.

What are some other reactions that Zephyr's boss could have?

_____

_____

_____

Now that you're aware of these two thinking traps, thinking back to the stressful situation that you described on Worksheet 8.2: Identifying and Evaluating Automatic Thoughts, which of the two types of common thinking traps (or both) best fits your automatic thought of that situation?

Flexible Thinking Can Overcome Stressful Automatic Thoughts

At this point, you should feel very proud of yourself! You waded through many heavy topics and feelings. You identified your unhelpful automatic thoughts and the impact they can have on your mental health. Now it's time to figure out how to change those pesky automatic thoughts.

Once our core beliefs are turned on by a triggering situation, we unfortunately tend to ignore information that would challenge those beliefs and focus only on what confirms them. Luckily, the rest of this chapter teaches some skills for helping you identify your core beliefs and develop more flexible ways of thinking.

One way to challenge unhelpful automatic thoughts is by being more *flexible* with our thoughts. This doesn't mean that we get rid of our automatic thoughts. Instead, we can allow our automatic thought to exist as one possible explanation, while also coming up with other possible interpretations.

Before you try being flexible with your own thoughts, let's see what this looks like in action with Andal, Elka, and Zephyr.

Andal was upset when their friends didn't invite them out. They automatically thought, "My friends don't like me. I'm annoying and inadequate." This left them feeling a lot of negative emotions. After being flexible with their thoughts, Andal came up with several other explanations:

1. I am a good friend; I had nothing to do with my friends' decision.
2. My friends happened to run into each other and it wasn't planned.
3. My friends texted me, but I didn't get the message.
4. If my friends didn't invite me out on purpose or think I'm not "trans enough," I deserve better from people I call my friends.

After being more flexible, Andal noticed that they felt freer and calmer knowing that there were a lot of different possible explanations and that their first negative thoughts weren't necessarily *the truth*.

Elka was stressed out after thinking about starting a conversation with a potential date. Her automatic thoughts were, "She wouldn't be interested in me. I would make a fool of myself." Thinking more flexibly, Elka came up with three new interpretations:

1. I have a lot to offer and someone would be lucky to date me.
2. Despite being nervous, I *can* talk to someone I'm interested in.
3. Even if I were to say or do something silly, everyone makes mistakes and it's not the end of the world.

After coming up with these explanations, Elka felt more confident and planned to talk to someone she's interested in.

When **Zephyr** felt anxious about telling their employer they were non-binary, they automatically thought, "My boss won't support me. Everything at work will be worse." They even went on to think they couldn't get a promotion in the future. Thinking more flexibly, Zephyr came up with three other explanations:

1. If I ask for support from my boss, she may respond positively.
2. Being honest with my boss might make work a more comfortable place for me.
3. Even if my boss is disrespectful, I am more confident that my coworkers will be respectful.

As a result, Zephyr felt more empowered about asking for what they need.

Andal, Elka, and Zephyr may seem like pros at being flexible and creating alternatives, but they had to learn and practice this skill—just like anyone would need to practice an instrument or sport to get good at it. It certainly did not come naturally to them.

When they first learned to be flexible with their thoughts, they found the questions in Box 8.1 to be helpful for coming up with alternative interpretations of stressful situations.

These questions are designed to help you get your thinking unstuck, to make it more flexible. Your responses to these questions can make it easier to come up with other possible interpretations. You may find it helpful to type these questions into your phone or take a picture of them so it's easier to use them in the future.

Now that you know what being flexible looks like *and* you have some questions to help you, it's time to practice what you've learned!

Using Worksheet 8.2: Identifying and Evaluating Automatic Thoughts, come up with *at least three* alternative explanations to counter the automatic interpretation you had in the stressful situation that you described on that worksheet. You can write them in the last column of the worksheet.

Now write down how these alternative explanations make you feel. How might being more flexible with your thoughts be useful to you?

_____

_____

_____

If you're anything like Andal, Elka, and Zephyr, your alternative explanations made you feel more positive, confident, and maybe even empowered compared to how your automatic interpretation made you feel. On the other hand, maybe you just feel less negative, anxious, or depressed than before (it's still a stressful situation after all!).

Keep in mind that feeling anxious, depressed, or uncertain is a normal response to stress. The goal of being flexible is not to remove all of your negative feelings and replace them with positive ones. Rather, the goal is to help you have more balanced, self-empowering thoughts when dealing with stressful situations.

Flexible thinking also comes in handy when dealing with LGBTQ-related stress. In addition to using the questions we discussed in Box 8.1, there are several skills that help us handle LGBTQ-related stress.

First, we can look at the anti-LGBTQ experience and think about whether it is:

(a) a real threat,
(b) something worth spending our time and energy on, and
(c) intended to hurt us.

Second, we can attribute anti-LGBTQ stress to ignorance by realizing that the individual(s) are ignorant, clueless, misinformed, and/or insensitive.

Third, we can tell ourselves that the situation is often temporary, and the situation will improve.

For instance, Eric was walking down the street holding his partner's hand. A man walked past, shook his head, and Eric heard him say, "Disgusting" under his breath. Eric's automatic thought about the situation was, "He's disgusting for saying that! I should teach him a lesson." But, because Eric wanted to be more flexible with his thoughts, he realized that, although ignorant, this guy did not pose a real threat to Eric and his partner's safety, and it was not something worth spending his time and energy on.

Eric's flexible thinking helped him to consider the facts of the situation, rather than resort to seeing only his automatic thought. His flexible thinking allowed him to blame the negative situation on the man's ignorance, rather than on something bad about himself. In the end, Eric felt good about himself because he prevented a worse outcome from potentially happening (e.g., getting hurt in a fight). Additionally, in the past, Eric would have thought about this experience for several days, but now he is able to more quickly let it go because it had nothing to do with who he is as a person. Importantly, this exercise does not question the reality of stigmatizing experiences or the harm they can do, but rather focuses on the ways these stigmatizing experiences can shape your thoughts and lead to internalized negative assumptions, especially about yourself, that can lead to depression, anxiety, or other distressing feelings.

Some Important Notes

First, it is important to note that fears of rejection may actually be realistic for LGBTQ people in some situations. To distinguish between realistic danger and expectations of rejection based on unhelpful ways of thinking learned from past experiences, ask yourself, "Am I responding based on my past experiences and biases or am I truly in danger in this situation?"

Second, as you grow more aware of your automatic thoughts, it is important to do so in a nonjudgmental way. Notice the thought and allow it to pass through your mind, rather than holding onto it. The goal is to be aware of the automatic thought and to see it as only one way of thinking about the situation. This will help you be more flexible in your thinking.

Finally, it is important to remind yourself that unhelpful automatic thoughts are not due to something bad about you—many are due to living in a society that often holds negative and stigmatizing views about LGBTQ people. In fact, you, and the entire LGBTQ community, possess remarkable strengths for coping with difficult situations!

Summary

Our past experiences drive us to form core beliefs. These core beliefs, in turn, influence the ways we automatically interpret situations around us. Noticing your automatic thoughts can be difficult at first, but within this chapter you have learned ways to identify unhelpful thinking—and how these thinking patterns can be formed over a lifetime of experiencing LGBTQ-related stress. Indeed, minority stress can lead to negative and harmful internalized thoughts about ourselves. You have learned that you can become more flexible with your thoughts by questioning them. This practice of identifying and challenging your most common and most rigid automatic thoughts can help you to develop greater flexibility in future situations—and, over time, to experience better mental health as well.

Home Practice: Identifying, Testing, and Changing Your Automatic Thoughts

Now it's time to put your new thinking skills to work! Think of this as "practice"—just like with sports, school, or hobbies, we only get better if we practice. If you get frustrated, that's OK—practice can be hard! Feel free to take a break. It can help to try out different times to work on the exercises until you find the time that works for you. Again, *regular* practice is more important than doing it "perfectly."

This week, practice identifying any automatic thoughts you have in response to stressful situations. Use Worksheet 8.2: Identifying and Evaluating Automatic Thoughts to keep track of this practice. Once you identify your automatic thought, try to come up with as many new interpretations as you can by identifying your "thinking traps" in that situation and using the questions outlined in Box 8.1, including:

- If what you're thinking were true, what would that mean?
- Why does it matter?
- What would happen if this were true?
- What would happen next?

Instructions: The following items ask about depression. For each item, indicate the number for the answer that best describes your experience over the past week.

—1. In the past week, how often have you felt depressed?

0 = **No depression** in the past week.

1 = **Infrequent depression**. Felt depressed a few times.

2 = **Occasional depression**. Felt depressed as much of the time as not.

3 = **Frequent depression**. Felt depressed most of the time.

4 = **Constant depression**. Felt depressed all of the time.

—2. In the past week, when you have felt depressed, how intense or severe was your depression?

0 = **Little or None**: Depression was absent or barely noticeable.

1 = **Mild**: Depression was at a low level.

2 = **Moderate**: Depression was intense at times.

3 = **Severe**: Depression was intense much of the time.

4 = **Extreme**: Depression was overwhelming.

—3. In the past week, how often did you have difficulty engaging in or being interested in activities you normally enjoy because of depression?

0 = **None**: I had no difficulty engaging in or being interested in activities that I normally enjoy because of depression.

1 = **Infrequent**: A few times I had difficulty engaging in or being interested in activities that I normally enjoy because of depression. My lifestyle was not affected.

2 = **Occasional**: I had some difficulty engaging in or being interested in activities that I normally enjoy because of depression. My lifestyle has only changed in minor ways.

3 = **Frequent**: I have considerable difficulty engaging in or being interested in activities that I normally enjoy because of depression. I have made significant changes in my lifestyle because of being unable to become interested in activities I used to enjoy.

4 = **All the Time**: I have been unable to participate in or be interested in activities that I normally enjoy because of depression. My lifestyle has been extensively affected and I no longer do things that I used to enjoy.

—4. In the past week, how much did your depression interfere with your ability to do the things you needed to do at work, at school, or at home?

0 = **None**: No interference at work/home/school from depression.

1 = **Mild**: My depression has caused some interference at work/home/school. Things are more difficult, but everything that needs to be done is still getting done.

2 = **Moderate**: My depression definitely interferes with tasks. Most things are still getting done, but few things are being done as well as in the past.

3 = **Severe**: My depression has really changed my ability to get things done. Some tasks are still being done, but many things are not. My performance has definitely suffered.

4 = **Extreme**: My depression has become incapacitating. I am unable to complete tasks and have had to leave school, have quit or been fired from my job, or have been unable to complete tasks at home and have faced consequences like bill collectors, eviction, etc.

—5. In the past week, how much has depression interfered with your social life and relationships?

0 = **None**: My depression doesn't affect my relationships.

1 = **Mild**: My depression slightly interferes with my relationships. Some of my friendships and other relationships have suffered, but, overall, my social life is still fulfilling.

2 = **Moderate**: I have experienced some interference with my social life, but I still have a few close relationships. I don't spend as much time with others as in the past, but I still socialize sometimes.

3 = **Severe**: My friendships and other relationships have suffered a lot because of depression. I do not enjoy social activities. I socialize very little.

4 = **Extreme**: My depression has completely disrupted my social activities. All of my relationships have suffered or ended. My family life is extremely strained.

Total Score: ___

Overall Anxiety Severity and Interference Scale (OASIS)

Instructions: The following items ask about anxiety and fear. For each item, indicate the number for the answer that best describes your experience over the past week.

—1. In the past week, how often have you felt anxious?

0 = **No anxiety** in the past week.

1 = **Infrequent anxiety.** Felt anxious a few times.

2 = **Occasional anxiety.** Felt anxious as much of the time as not. It was hard to relax.

3 = **Frequent anxiety.** Felt anxious most of the time. It was very difficult to relax.

4 = **Constant anxiety.** Felt anxious all of the time and never really relaxed.

—2. In the past week, when you have felt anxious, how intense or severe was your anxiety?

0 = **Little or None:** Anxiety was absent or barely noticeable.

1 = **Mild:** Anxiety was at a low level. It was possible to relax when I tried. Physical symptoms were only slightly uncomfortable.

2 = **Moderate:** Anxiety was distressing at times. It was hard to relax or concentrate, but I could do it if I tried. Physical symptoms were uncomfortable.

3 = **Severe:** Anxiety was intense much of the time. It was very difficult to relax or focus on anything else. Physical symptoms were extremely uncomfortable.

4 = **Extreme:** Anxiety was overwhelming. It was impossible to relax at all. Physical symptoms were unbearable.

—3. In the past week, how often did you avoid situations, places, objects, or activities because of anxiety or fear?

0 = **None:** I do not avoid places, situations, activities, or things because of fear.

1 = **Infrequent:** I avoid something once in a while, but will usually face the situation or confront the object. My lifestyle is not affected.

2 = **Occasional:** I have some fear of certain situations, places, or objects, but it is still manageable. My lifestyle has only changed in minor ways. I always or almost always avoid the things I fear when I'm alone, but can handle them if someone comes with me.

3 = **Frequent:** I have considerable fear and really try to avoid the things that frighten me. I have made significant changes in my lifestyle to avoid the object, situation, activity, or place.

4 = **All the Time:** Avoiding objects, situations, activities, or places has taken over my life. My lifestyle has been extensively affected and I no longer do things that I used to enjoy.

—4. In the past week, how much did your anxiety interfere with your ability to do the things you needed to do at work, at school, or at home?

0 = **None:** No interference at work/home/school from anxiety.

1 = **Mild:** My anxiety has caused some interference at work/home/school. Things are more difficult, but everything that needs to be done is still getting done.

2 = **Moderate:** My anxiety definitely interferes with tasks. Most things are still getting done, but few things are being done as well as in the past.

3 = **Severe:** My anxiety has really changed my ability to get things done. Some tasks are still being done, but many things are not. My performance has definitely suffered.

4 = **Extreme:** My anxiety has become incapacitating. I am unable to complete tasks and have had to leave school, have quit or been fired from my job, or have been unable to complete tasks at home and have faced consequences like bill collectors, eviction, etc.

—5. In the past week, how much has anxiety interfered with your social life and relationships?

0 = **None:** My anxiety doesn't affect my relationships.

1 = **Mild:** My anxiety slightly interferes with my relationships. Some of my friendships and other relationships have suffered, but, overall, my social life is still fulfilling.

2 = **Moderate:** I have experienced some interference with my social life, but I still have a few close relationships. I don't spend as much time with others as in the past, but I still socialize sometimes.

3 = **Severe:** My friendships and other relationships have suffered a lot because of anxiety. I do not enjoy social activities. I socialize very little.

4 = **Extreme:** My anxiety has completely disrupted my social activities. All of my relationships have suffered or ended. My family life is extremely strained.

Total Score: ___

Progress Record

ODSIS

```
20 ─────────────────────────────────────────
18 ─────────────────────────────────────────
16 ─────────────────────────────────────────
14 ─────────────────────────────────────────
12 ─────────────────────────────────────────
10 ─────────────────────────────────────────
 8 ─────────────────────────────────────────
 6 ─────────────────────────────────────────
 4 ─────────────────────────────────────────
 2 ─────────────────────────────────────────
 0 ─────────────────────────────────────────
```

| Week 1 | 2 | 3 | 4 | 5 | 6 | 7 | 8 | 9 | 10 | 11 | 12 | 13 | 14 | 15 | 16 | 17 | 18 | 19 | 20 | 21 | 22 | 23 | 24 | v |

OASIS

```
20 ─────────────────────────────────────────
18 ─────────────────────────────────────────
16 ─────────────────────────────────────────
14 ─────────────────────────────────────────
12 ─────────────────────────────────────────
10 ─────────────────────────────────────────
 8 ─────────────────────────────────────────
 6 ─────────────────────────────────────────
 4 ─────────────────────────────────────────
 2 ─────────────────────────────────────────
 0 ─────────────────────────────────────────
```

| Week 1 | 2 | 3 | 4 | 5 | 6 | 7 | 8 | 9 | 10 | 11 | 12 | 13 | 14 | 15 | 16 | 17 | 18 | 19 | 20 | 21 | 22 | 23 | 24 | v |

Other Assessment

```
20 ─────────────────────────────────────────
18 ─────────────────────────────────────────
16 ─────────────────────────────────────────
14 ─────────────────────────────────────────
12 ─────────────────────────────────────────
10 ─────────────────────────────────────────
 8 ─────────────────────────────────────────
 6 ─────────────────────────────────────────
 4 ─────────────────────────────────────────
 2 ─────────────────────────────────────────
 0 ─────────────────────────────────────────
```

| Week 1 | 2 | 3 | 4 | 5 | 6 | 7 | 8 | 9 | 10 | 11 | 12 | 13 | 14 | 15 | 16 | 17 | 18 | 19 | 20 | 21 | 22 | 23 | 24 | v |

Worksheet 8.1: Downward Arrow Technique

Automatic Interpretation:

_____

⬇

If this were true, what would it mean about me? Why does this matter to me?
What would happen if this were true? What would happen next?

Underlying Interpretation:

_____

⬇

If this were true, what would it mean about me? Why does this matter to me?
What would happen if this were true? What would happen next?

Underlying Interpretation:

_____

⬇

If this were true, what would it mean about me? Why does this matter to me?
What would happen if this were true? What would happen next?

Underlying Interpretation:

_____

⬇

If this were true, what would it mean about me? Why does this matter to me?
What would happen if this were true? What would happen next?

Underlying Interpretation:

_____

Example: *Some friends went out last night without inviting me.*

Automatic Interpretation: *I knew they never really liked me*

If this were true, what would it mean about me? Why does this matter to me?
What would happen if this were true? What would happen next?

Underlying Interpretation: *They rejected me because I'm awkward and not fun to hang out with. And I've always known I'm not "trans enough" for them.*

If this were true, what would it mean about me? Why does this matter to me?
What would happen if this were true? What would happen next?

Underlying Interpretation: *If what I wrote were true, it would mean that there's nothing to like about me.*

If this were true, what would it mean about me? Why does this matter to me?
What would happen if this were true? What would happen next?

Underlying Interpretation: *It would mean that I'll never fit in.*

If this were true, what would it mean about me? Why does this matter to me?
What would happen if this were true? What would happen next?

Underlying Interpretation : *It would mean that I'm unlovable.*

Figure 8.2

Downward Arrow Technique—LGBTQ-Related Stress Example

Worksheet 8.2: Identifying and Evaluating Automatic Thoughts

Situation/Trigger	Automatic Thought(s) or Interpretations(s)	Emotions(s)	Identify "Thinking Trap"	Generate Alternative Thoughts(s) or Interpretation(s)

Situation/ Trigger	Automatic Thought(s) or Interpretation(s)	Emotion(s)	Identify "Thinking Trap"	Generate Alternative Thought(s) or Interpretation(s)
Called a friend in the morning and haven't heard back yet.	She doesn't like me. She thinks I'm annoying.	Ashamed, alone, self-conscious	Jumping to conclusions	1. She's busy and hasn't heard my message yet. 2. Her phone died.
Saw another queer woman of color at a party and am interested.	If I introduce myself, I'm going to make a fool of myself and they will reject me and make fun of me. I won't be able to handle it.	Anxious, afraid, embarrassed	Thinking the worst	1. They may not reject me. 2. I've been rejected before and survived.
Boss asked to meet with me later today	She doesn't like my work. I'm going to get fired. I'm a failure and the worst person.	Anxious, tense, afraid	Thinking the worst	1. She may want to review my work or a new project. 2. I usually get good feedback and perform well during our meetings.
An attractive guy asks me out	He won't like me when we actually go out. I'm not good-looking enough, fit enough, or smart enough. I have to work really hard tonight at getting him to like me.	Insecure, pressured, afraid	Jumping to conclusions	1. He asked me out, so he's clearly interested. 2. I'm a good person with much to offer. 3. No one is perfect.
A feminine, flamboyant gay male coworker is talking about his weekend	He's so flamboyant, feminine, and annoying. People will think I'm like that too. People don't like gays because of feminine gay guys like him.	Uncomfortable, anxious, annoyed	Jumping to conclusions	1. He's just expressing himself. I also want to be accepted for who I am. 2. He has the right to express himself how he wants. 3. Others may not find him annoying.
Saw a politician on TV condemning trans people	I have to work extra hard to show transphobic people that I'm just as good as they are, if not better than them.	Tense, angry	Thinking the worst	1. Even if some people won't accept me for being trans, others accept me just the way I am.

Figure 8.3

Identifying and Evaluating Automatic Thoughts—LGBTQ-Related Stress Examples

Module 6: Countering Emotional Behaviors

Chapter 9 Overview

In this chapter you will learn how your emotions can drive your behaviors. These behaviors are called *emotional behaviors* and usually serve important functions. For example, emotional behaviors often reduce how intense an emotion is and can even help us survive difficult situations. However, some emotional behaviors may be less helpful and even harmful when used all the time or in certain contexts.

This chapter will help you identify situations, activities, and people that lead you to use unhelpful emotional behaviors. It will also help you to develop different behaviors for distressing situations to improve your mood, relationships, and self-esteem so that emotional behaviors can start losing the power they currently have on your life.

Chapter 9 Outline

- Weekly Check-In
- Review Home Practice from Chapter 8
- What Are Emotional Behaviors?
- Emotional Behaviors and LGBTQ-Related Stress
- What Are Your Emotional Behaviors?
- Emotional Behaviors Are a Paradox!
- The Pros and Cons of Emotional Behaviors

Weekly Check-In

Take a minute to track your symptoms using the ODSIS and OASIS, located at the end of this chapter. You may also photocopy these forms or download multiple copies by searching for this book's title on the Oxford Academic platform at academic.oup.com. Do you notice any changes? What do you attribute these changes to?

Review Home Practice from Chapter 8

How did it go with identifying and challenging your automatic thoughts, the home practice for Chapter 8? If you had difficulties, don't worry—this is normal. Most people don't "master" this skill the first time (or even the first several times) they try it. It takes practice for this process of challenging unhelpful thoughts to feel normal and natural.

Here are some tricks to help you keep practicing and working towards building this skill of identifying and challenging unhelpful thoughts:

- Keep using your mindful self-awareness skill to slow down your thoughts when experiencing strong emotions. Refer back to Chapter 7 (Module 4: Increasing Mindful Awareness of LGBTQ-Related Stress Reactions) for a reminder of how slowing down will give you a chance to notice and challenge your unhelpful thoughts.
- Even if you "miss the opportunity" to identify and challenge unhelpful thoughts in the moment, you can still practice after the fact. It's never too late to do this!
- If you're working with a therapist, let them know you are having difficulty with this skill; they can help you to continue practicing in your sessions.

Emotional behaviors refers to the things we do to manage our emotions. This includes things we do to (1) avoid feeling strong emotions, (2) keep emotions from getting too intense, and (3) stop strong emotions from continuing once they have started.

Because we live in a society that often holds negative, stigmatizing views of LGBTQ people, it's common to have had painful experiences, like being bullied or rejected. These experiences can make LGBTQ people feel strong, negative emotions, like anger or worthlessness. These emotions can be overwhelming and difficult to manage at times, and it is common to start avoiding them, trying to prevent them, or finding ways to reduce them once they start.

Sometimes these behaviors can actually be helpful. For example, earlier in this workbook, you learned that sadness often prompts people to withdraw or work through a loss or setback. Anger motivates people to defend themselves when they've been wronged. Anxiety helps people to prepare for important future events. However, sometimes emotional behaviors are not so helpful. Here are some examples of emotional behaviors that are unhelpful:

- In Mia's case, self-harm is an emotional behavior. Mia harmed herself to manage powerful emotions that she didn't know how to handle. Not only did self-harm cause physical harm to Mia's body, but it also hurt her relationships.
- For Ben, sex is an emotional behavior. Although sex is good and healthy, the way Ben was using it actually caused problems in his life, like missed appointments and less time with family and friends. He used sex to avoid the feelings of sadness and rejection, but sex only made those feelings more intense.
- Salvador's emotional behaviors are distraction and unassertiveness. His family regularly says things like, "Thank God none of our kids are gay!" Although Salvador feels angry about this, he can't say anything because he is afraid of being found out. He also feels like he doesn't fit in at school and feels sad and lonely. To cope, Salvador stays quiet when his family makes a derogatory comment and distracts himself by watching TV or reading all the time.

Just like Mia, Ben, and Salvador, we all act in ways that reduce distress and make us feel better in the short term. These emotional behaviors might feel like a release from the tension you're feeling, but the relief is often short-lived, and these behaviors can make you feel worse later. For Mia, Ben, and Salvador, their emotional behaviors ultimately led to strained relationships, physical harm, chronic unassertiveness, and increased negative emotions.

What kinds of things do you think you do to (1) avoid feeling strong emotions, (2) keep emotions from getting too intense, and (3) stop strong emotions from continuing after they've already started? You can also use Worksheet 9.1: List of Emotional Behaviors, located at the end of this chapter, to track these emotional behaviors. You may also download a copy of the worksheet by searching for this book's title on the Oxford Academic platform at academic.oup.com.

As you'll see in the worksheet, we generally think of three kinds of emotional behaviors: (1) behavioral avoidance—which can be subtle or overt, (2) cognitive avoidance, and (3) using safety signals. Let's go through each one and see how they relate to your experiences.

Behavioral Avoidance

Behavioral avoidance includes any *behaviors* that you do that help you feel better when you are experiencing strong emotions. This might include, for example, pacing, biting your nails, scrolling through social media, having sex, or using drugs.

Leslie gets very nervous whenever she's in social situations. She knows that when she gets really nervous, she starts to shake. She keeps her anxiety under control by avoiding eye contact, focusing on breathing deeply, and drinking alcohol. When she does these three things, she prevents her anxiety from getting so bad that she shakes.

What are some *behaviors* you use to avoid or stop intense emotions? These behaviors could be really subtle and hard to notice (e.g., always wearing sunglasses to avoid others' judgment) or overt and obvious (e.g., declining a date simply to avoid rejection). Write them down here:

_____

_____

_____

Cognitive Avoidance

Cognitive avoidance includes any *mental techniques* that you use to feel better when you are in a situation you cannot leave. This might include distracting yourself (by watching TV or listening to music), "tuning out" of a conversation, or trying to think of something other than the current situation.

Brendan plays on the college soccer team. His teammates are mostly conservative, homophobic men who don't know he is gay. They make a lot of anti-LGBTQ comments and jokes, which makes Brendan angry. When he gets angry, he gets hot and sweaty and turns red. Brendan thinks that if his teammates noticed this, he would out himself. He stops himself from getting angry by making himself think about things that make him happy, like walking on his favorite beach or playing with his dog, and avoiding any negative thoughts, like how insensitive his teammates are.

What are some mental techniques you use to avoid or stop intense emotions? Write these down here:

_____

_____

_____

Safety Signals

Safety signals include *anything that you carry with you, or that you do before going out,* that makes you feel more comfortable. This could include carrying a water bottle or medication, wearing sunglasses or hats, or carrying the name of your doctor or other important people.

Sheena always makes sure to carry her phone and something to read in case she ever gets into awkward situations, like strangers wanting to talk to her. If she didn't have her phone and book, she is certain she wouldn't be able to handle this.

What are some safety signals you use to avoid or prevent intense emotions? Write down your safety signals here:

_____

_____

_____

Emotional behaviors often come from stressful experiences, including anti-LGBTQ experiences and LGBTQ-related stress. To help you understand this, let's think about Leslie, Brendan, and Sheena, discussed above:

- Leslie gets very anxious in social situations. She avoids eye contact, focuses on deep breaths, and drinks alcohol to make her feel safe and in control (behavioral avoidance). Looking back, when Leslie was young, she was bullied because she presented as gender nonconforming. This made her feel ashamed and like she didn't "fit in." Now, as a young adult, these same emotions come up in social situations, so she uses similar strategies to feel safe.

- Because he always played on homophobic soccer teams, Brendan has dealt with anti-LGBTQ experiences since he was a kid. By avoiding any negative thoughts (cognitive avoidance), he kept himself safe and in control as a kid and now.

- Today Sheena carries her phone and book to help her feel safe and in control in situations where she might feel inferior. Because Sheena was made to feel inferior and worthless about her gender identity as a child, she uses safety signals to feel comfortable when she's out alone.

Another common example of how emotional behaviors are related to LGBTQ-related stress is if you think about sex and substances as potential emotional behaviors. For example:

- Anti-LGBTQ experiences can make LGBTQ people feel unloved and unwanted. It's not uncommon to learn to use sex as a way of dealing with these overwhelming negative emotions and experiences.

- In general, everyone has different standards for their own sexual behaviors, and through this treatment you'll learn to recognize for yourself when sex in your life happens in fun, enjoyable, and safe contexts, and when it's used to avoid negative emotions.

- Using sex to avoid negative emotions takes away from the healthy and useful aspects of sex, including stress relief (i.e., in fun and enjoyable contexts, as a positive part of LGBTQ individuals' lives) and feeling loved.

- Using sex to avoid negative emotions can actually end up making us feel worse about ourselves.

- Alcohol and other drug use, with or without sex, can have a similar effect on our self-esteem. For example, Sam drinks beer before sex to avoid internalized negative (and inaccurate) thoughts that sex between men is "dirty" or "dangerous." Drinking alcohol before sex helps Sam relax and enjoy sex with other men more. However, afterwards, he ends up feeling more ashamed and hopeless.
- At the same time, using alcohol or drugs safely and in moderation can be a fun and social activity for some people in some contexts. Throughout this treatment, you'll come to identify in what situations using substances represents an emotional behavior for you.

What Are Your Emotional Behaviors?

Looking at the emotional behaviors you listed on Worksheet 9.1, how do you think they might be related to early or ongoing experiences of LGBTQ-related stress? Write down some potential origins of your emotional behaviors here:

_____

_____

_____

In comparison to heterosexual or cisgender people, LGBTQ people may have more challenges identifying their emotional behaviors because of their experiences learning that their emotions are bad, wrong, or shameful. Using Box 9.1, let's try another way of identifying your emotional behaviors, this time in response to specific emotions. Write down the emotional behavior that you did (or were tempted to do or that you avoided doing) in response to each of the listed emotions.

Was it hard to identify behaviors that go along with your emotions? If so, sometimes it is easier to start with the behavior that felt unhelpful to you and think back to what you were feeling or experiencing before you did that behavior. Let's try that, using Table 9.1.

What did you notice? Were you able to make a connection between your emotions and a behavior that came after?

Sometimes an emotional behavior can be a lack of behavior. For example, many LGBTQ people commonly avoid strong emotions because of a long history of being in threatening situations (e.g., transphobic comments,

Box 9.1. Connecting Emotions and Emotional Behaviors

Think back to the last time you felt each of the following emotions.

- When you felt each of the specific emotions in the left column, what did you do? What were you tempted to do? Did you feel an automatic urge to behave in any particular way?
- Write that behavior under each emotion below.

Emotion	Emotional Behavior
Anxiety	
Guilt	
Happiness	
Loneliness	
Other emotions:	

invalidating and discriminatory laws and policies). These avoidance behaviors might include avoiding close connections with others, being a perfectionist at school or work, avoiding social situations, or not standing up for yourself.

Identifying emotional behaviors can be difficult if you aren't used to identifying your emotions. But by using your mindful awareness skills, you can better understand how your emotions drive your actions.

Table 9.1. Tracing Unhelpful (Emotional) Behaviors Back to Their Origin

Unhelpful Behavior from the Past Week	What You Were Feeling Right Before the Unhelpful Behavior

Emotional behaviors are avoidant—they help (in the short term) to prevent, avoid, and reduce uncomfortable emotions. To help you understand how avoiding your emotions can be problematic, let's try an experiment! You will need a timer to complete this experiment.

Let's get started! First, set your timer for 60 seconds.

Now, for the next 60 seconds, do **not** think about a stressful anti-LGBTQ experience that you've had. You can think about anything else you want; just don't think about any anti-LGBTQ experiences that you've had.

Go!

What was this experience like for you? What did you think about? How often did you think about anti-LGBTQ experiences you've had? You probably thought about at least one anti-LGBTQ experience you've had. This happens because when people try to **not** think about something, trying to push down or avoid the thought actually increases the chance of thinking about the very thing you're trying not to think about!

This exercise shows how trying to avoid or push away thoughts and emotions tends to backfire. Pushing away thoughts and emotions can even make them *more* frequent and intense. And even if you are able to push them away for a short time, you will probably have to "check" to make sure these thoughts or memories are not in your mind. Doing this involves thinking about the memory or situation. So, pushing away thoughts and emotions makes you think about them more, AND increases the number of times you'll think about them.

Let's try something different. This time, **think** about a specific unpleasant anti-LGBTQ experience that you've had and keep this in mind until your strong emotions in response to it eventually fade.

What was this like for you? What happened to your negative emotions? Did they eventually fade? Write about your experience here:

_____

_____

_____

Thinking of the emotional behaviors you've identified so far, what do you think are some of the benefits (pros) and costs (cons) of using them in your life? List these in Table 9.2.

Looking at the pros you listed in Table 9.2, it's clear that emotional behaviors can be really useful in the short term: You can immediately avoid feeling anxious, uneasy, or upset in stressful situations. Unfortunately, emotional behaviors have a lot of downsides in the long run, and using them can actually make problems worse:

1. Emotional behaviors stop you from *habituating* to a situation. Habituation means that the more times you face a feared situation and stay in it, the less stressed out by it you'll feel over time. *For instance, the first time Sam had sex without drinking, he experienced really intense anxious feelings. However, over time, as he continued to have sex without drinking, his anxious feelings were less intense and went away more quickly. Eventually, he realized that he no longer had negative or anxious feelings when he had sex with other men.*

2. Emotion avoidance stops you from feeling *in control* of the situation and learning that you can handle it. *For example, Sam drank beer*

Table 9.2. Pros and Cons of Your Emotional Behaviors

+ Pros of your emotional behaviors	
- Cons of your emotional behaviors	

before having sex because he didn't think he would be able to handle his negative emotions otherwise. While drinking made him feel better in the short term, it strengthened his belief that he couldn't handle his negative emotions without alcohol and made it more likely that he would drink before having sex the next time. As part of this program, Sam tried having sex without drinking. Over time Sam had sex without drinking a few times. Soon he noticed that he felt more in control of his negative emotions because he knew he could handle them without having to rely on drinking.

3. Emotion avoidance stops you from *challenging your automatic interpretations* about situations and developing more accurate beliefs. *For instance, Sam's automatic interpretation about having sex without drinking was that he would be so anxious that he wouldn't be able to enjoy sex. But after having sex without drinking many times, his negative feelings went away and he was able to enjoy sex. This showed him that his automatic interpretation was wrong. Ultimately, experiencing his emotions instead of avoiding them gave him more control over his day-to-day life. The same can happen for you!*

Earlier in this workbook, you learned about mindfulness and present-focused awareness as tools to help you feel less overwhelmed by your emotions. Using these tools to focus on your primary emotions in the moment will help you listen and respond to the important messages they are telling you.

Why Do You Keep Doing These Emotional Behaviors If They Are So Bad for You?

As we said earlier, unhelpful emotional behaviors provide short-term relief from distress. When a behavior makes you feel better, even just for a little while, you are more likely to do it again. Think of it like this: If you were in a great deal of physical pain and pushing a button administered pain medication that made you feel better, you'd probably keep pushing it. Immediate reinforcement, like feeling relief right after an emotional behavior, is really difficult to break—even when we know that it will backfire in the long term.

As you just learned, when you enter a situation that brings up a strong emotion, the urge to do something that "worked" (reduced the negative emotions quickly) can be very strong. For example:

Samantha often avoids going on dates when she gets asked out because dating makes her feel panicky. When she turns down a date, her panicky feelings go away. So, she keeps turning down dates, and never asks anyone out. And why would she? Who wants to feel panicky!? But this is really taking a toll on Samantha: She would like to be in a relationship one day and is losing hope that this could happen.

Although avoiding dates makes Samantha feel better in the moment, her avoidance of dating also reinforces her negative beliefs. In some ways, she is, to herself, confirming her beliefs that dating and romantic connections are dangerous. In that moment, her automatic thought was that the only reason she didn't panic was because she avoided the date. But avoiding uncomfortable emotions, like anxiety and panic, makes those emotions stronger. And yes, Samantha has noticed that over time, getting asked out has made her feel even more anxious than before, and now just thinking about the possibility of going on a date makes her feel panicky.

Just like Samantha, you might have emotional behaviors that quickly get rid of uncomfortable emotions in the short term. To change this pattern, it can be helpful to understand both the short- and long-term results of your emotional behaviors. Let's think about situations that made *you* feel strong emotions and examine what happened in response.

First, take a recent situation in which you were feeling strong emotions. What was the situation? What emotions were you experiencing? Take a moment to identify the specific behaviors that were prompted or "driven" by the emotions. Remember to include more subtle behaviors. Write these down below:

Situation:

_____

_____

_____

Emotions:

_____

_____

_____

Emotional behaviors:

_____

_____

_____

Now, let's look at how to potentially start breaking this cycle. Take a close look at the behaviors you just listed to answer the following questions (space to write down your answers is provided below):

- What was the purpose or *function* of these emotional behaviors (what did the behavior do)?
    - Do they seem reasonable and helpful, given the nature of the situation?
    - How did engaging in these behaviors make you feel?
- What were the short-term results of these behaviors?
- What were the long-term results of these behaviors?
- How would you have liked to act differently in response to your emotions?

Function of emotional behaviors:

_____

_____

_____

Short-term results:

_____

_____

_____

Long-term results:

_____

_____

_____

How would you have liked to act differently in response to your emotions?

_____

_____

_____

When considering the function of your emotional behaviors, you are likely to find that these strategies only really helped reduce your negative emotions in the short term. But what happens in the long term? When you escape situations that frighten you, it's normal to feel a temporary sense of relief. You might wipe your brow and think to yourself, "Phew, I got out of there just in time." But what happens the next time you go back into that situation? Will you be more or less afraid?

Remember, you're not here to learn ways to control or push away your emotions. That's because strategies to control or push away emotions will most likely end up making the very emotions you are trying to avoid feel more intense and stick around longer. Instead, the goal of this treatment program is to learn how to fully experience, accept, and tolerate your full range of emotions, and to learn to respond to your emotional experiences more flexibly.

How to Break the Cycle

You might feel overwhelmed when you notice how often you use emotional behaviors. Most people have emotional behaviors that cause them distress. You are not alone, and emotional behaviors can be changed!

One of the best ways to break this cycle is to learn how to replace a current emotional behavior with a new, more helpful behavior (even though this is difficult). For example, when you're feeling sad, even if you don't feel like it *at all*, you could try to text your friends instead of taking a nap. Approaching your emotions instead of avoiding them is important in order to learn about your ability to cope in a given situation. Another example: If you always avoid crowds out of fear that you will have a panic attack, you will assume you cannot handle being in a crowd. But if you approach the situation, and go into a crowd on purpose, you could learn more about how well you can manage.

For example:

Nish often has difficulty standing up for their needs, opinions, and preferences. They noticed that they usually do this to avoid rejection and avoid feeling inferior. Growing up, Nish was often rejected and made to feel inferior because they are gender nonconforming.

Let's pretend you are Nish's therapist. Nish tells you that when their girlfriend and her friends were talking about an upcoming party, Nish avoided telling her that they didn't want to go because there were going to be a lot of drugs there. What is a different way Nish could respond to this situation instead of not standing up for themselves? Write it below:

_____

_____

_____

Now let's consider one of the emotional behaviors *you* identified in the previous section. List it here:

_____

_____

_____

Can you think of a different way of responding when you feel the identified emotion? Write it here:

_____

_____

_____

Table 9.3. Emotional Behaviors and New Behaviors

Emotional Behavior	Possible LGBTQ-Related Stress Origins	New Behavior
Avoiding romantic connections with same-gender partners	Internalized stigma	Creating a profile on an LGBTQ-dating website
Being a perfectionist at school or work	Experiences of actual or feared rejection	Leaving things untidy or unfinished
Avoiding cisgender or heterosexual people	Experiences of actual or feared rejection; hiding your LGBTQ status	Asking a cisgender or heterosexual coworker out to lunch
Leaving a social situation	Fear of rejection; hiding your LGBTQ status	Staying in a situation and approaching people
Using alcohol or other drugs during sex	Fear of rejection; internalized stigma	Having sex without using alcohol or other drugs
Being on edge and always looking out for threats	Being the victim of anti-LGBTQ discrimination or violence; fears of rejection; hiding your LGBTQ status	Focusing attention on the current task; mindfulness

Sometimes it can be tough to think of new behaviors. If you find yourself getting stuck, maybe start by thinking of the most extreme opposite action that you can. For example, if someone's emotional behavior when feeling sad is to spend time alone, the most extreme opposite might be going to a concert or talking to every stranger they see.

Those behaviors might not be possible (or helpful). But by first thinking of extreme behaviors, you can then start scaling back to find a new behavior that works for you. Perhaps the person who avoids people when sad can talk to a stranger, or call a friend and suggest that they do something together. Thinking of the most extreme opposite can help you start to brainstorm.

Table 9.3 lists common emotional behaviors that many LGBTQ people experience, alongside some possible new behaviors. Maybe your own emotional behaviors and new behaviors are similar to something on this list.

You'll learn more about how to change emotional behaviors in future sessions, but for right now, just note some of the behaviors you would like to change. You can start tracking these on Worksheet 9.2: Alternative Action, which is located at the end of this chapter and also available for download by searching for this book's title on the Oxford Academic platform at academic.oup.com.

Summary

Today, you learned about how emotional behaviors develop and maintain themselves and can be linked to your LGBTQ-related stress experiences. You also learned how to challenge those emotional behaviors and try out new ones that may be challenging but also will likely get you closer to your goals. How you feel may not change right away, but over time, changing how you behave can also change how you feel. As you know, thoughts, bodily feelings, and behaviors come together to create our emotional experiences. Changing how you respond to one of those pieces can change your whole experience.

Home Practice: Identifying Alternative Actions

This week, practice identifying your emotional behaviors and alternative actions using Worksheet 9.2: Alternative Action. When you notice yourself engaging in an emotional behavior, try to think of a new behavior.

You don't need to start trying out the alternative behaviors (that will come in the next chapters), but if you have the opportunity and feel ready to try some out, go for it! You can even purposefully enter situations that would normally lead to an emotional behavior and experiment with trying out your alternative action, assuming these situations do not pose an actual threat. If you do start trying out your alternative actions, begin with situations that are only mildly emotionally distressing. You can build your way up to more intensely distressing situations over time.

Lastly, remember that this is practice, and it gets easier the more that you do it.

Overall Depression Severity and Interference Scale (ODSIS)

Instructions: The following items ask about depression. For each item, indicate the number for the answer that best describes your experience over the past week.

—1. In the past week, how often have you felt depressed?

0 = **No depression** in the past week.

1 = **Infrequent depression**. Felt depressed a few times.

2 = **Occasional depression**. Felt depressed as much of the time as not.

3 = **Frequent depression**. Felt depressed most of the time.

4 = **Constant depression**. Felt depressed all of the time.

—2. In the past week, when you have felt depressed, how intense or severe was your depression?

0 = **Little or None**: Depression was absent or barely noticeable.

1 = **Mild**: Depression was at a low level.

2 = **Moderate**: Depression was intense at times.

3 = **Severe**: Depression was intense much of the time.

4 = **Extreme**: Depression was overwhelming.

—3. In the past week, how often did you have difficulty engaging in or being interested in activities you normally enjoy because of depression?

0 = **None**: I had no difficulty engaging in or being interested in activities that I normally enjoy because of depression.

1 = **Infrequent**: A few times I had difficulty engaging in or being interested in activities that I normally enjoy because of depression. My lifestyle was not affected.

2 = **Occasional**: I had some difficulty engaging in or being interested in activities that I normally enjoy because of depression. My lifestyle has only changed in minor ways.

3 = **Frequent**: I have considerable difficulty engaging in or being interested in activities that I normally enjoy because of depression. I have made significant changes in my lifestyle because of being unable to become interested in activities I used to enjoy.

4 = **All the Time**: I have been unable to participate in or be interested in activities that I normally enjoy because of depression. My lifestyle has been extensively affected and I no longer do things that I used to enjoy.

—4. In the past week, how much did your depression interfere with your ability to do the things you needed to do at work, at school, or at home?

0 = **None**: No interference at work/home/school from depression.

1 = **Mild**: My depression has caused some interference at work/home/school. Things are more difficult, but everything that needs to be done is still getting done.

2 = **Moderate**: My depression definitely interferes with tasks. Most things are still getting done, but few things are being done as well as in the past.

3 = **Severe**: My depression has really changed my ability to get things done. Some tasks are still being done, but many things are not. My performance has definitely suffered.

4 = **Extreme**: My depression has become incapacitating. I am unable to complete tasks and have had to leave school, have quit or been fired from my job, or have been unable to complete tasks at home and have faced consequences like bill collectors, eviction, etc.

—5. In the past week, how much has depression interfered with your social life and relationships?

0 = **None**: My depression doesn't affect my relationships.

1 = **Mild**: My depression slightly interferes with my relationships. Some of my friendships and other relationships have suffered, but, overall, my social life is still fulfilling.

2 = **Moderate**: I have experienced some interference with my social life, but I still have a few close relationships. I don't spend as much time with others as in the past, but I still socialize sometimes.

3 = **Severe**: My friendships and other relationships have suffered a lot because of depression. I do not enjoy social activities. I socialize very little.

4 = **Extreme**: My depression has completely disrupted my social activities. All of my relationships have suffered or ended. My family life is extremely strained.

Total Score: ____

Overall Anxiety Severity and Interference Scale (OASIS)

Instructions: The following items ask about anxiety and fear. For each item, indicate the number for the answer that best describes your experience over the past week.

—1. In the past week, how often have you felt anxious?

  0 = **No anxiety** in the past week.

  1 = **Infrequent anxiety.** Felt anxious a few times.

  2 = **Occasional anxiety.** Felt anxious as much of the time as not. It was hard to relax.

  3 = **Frequent anxiety.** Felt anxious most of the time. It was very difficult to relax.

  4 = **Constant anxiety.** Felt anxious all of the time and never really relaxed.

—2. In the past week, when you have felt anxious, how intense or severe was your anxiety?

  0 = **Little or None:** Anxiety was absent or barely noticeable.

  1 = **Mild:** Anxiety was at a low level. It was possible to relax when I tried. Physical symptoms were only slightly uncomfortable.

  2 = **Moderate:** Anxiety was distressing at times. It was hard to relax or concentrate, but I could do it if I tried. Physical symptoms were uncomfortable.

  3 = **Severe:** Anxiety was intense much of the time. It was very difficult to relax or focus on anything else. Physical symptoms were extremely uncomfortable.

  4 = **Extreme:** Anxiety was overwhelming. It was impossible to relax at all. Physical symptoms were unbearable.

—3. In the past week, how often did you avoid situations, places, objects, or activities because of anxiety or fear?

  0 = **None:** I do not avoid places, situations, activities, or things because of fear.

  1 = **Infrequent:** I avoid something once in a while, but will usually face the situation or confront the object. My lifestyle is not affected.

  2 = **Occasional:** I have some fear of certain situations, places, or objects, but it is still manageable. My lifestyle has only changed in minor ways. I always or almost always avoid the things I fear when I'm alone, but can handle them if someone comes with me.

  3 = **Frequent:** I have considerable fear and really try to avoid the things that frighten me. I have made significant changes in my lifestyle to avoid the object, situation, activity, or place.

  4 = **All the Time:** Avoiding objects, situations, activities, or places has taken over my life. My lifestyle has been extensively affected and I no longer do things that I used to enjoy.

—4. In the past week, how much did your anxiety interfere with your ability to do the things you needed to do at work, at school, or at home?

  0 = **None:** No interference at work/home/school from anxiety.

  1 = **Mild:** My anxiety has caused some interference at work/home/school. Things are more difficult, but everything that needs to be done is still getting done.

2 = **Moderate:** My anxiety definitely interferes with tasks. Most things are still getting done, but few things are being done as well as in the past.

3 = **Severe:** My anxiety has really changed my ability to get things done. Some tasks are still being done, but many things are not. My performance has definitely suffered.

4 = **Extreme:** My anxiety has become incapacitating. I am unable to complete tasks and have had to leave school, have quit or been fired from my job, or have been unable to complete tasks at home and have faced consequences like bill collectors, eviction, etc.

—5. In the past week, how much has anxiety interfered with your social life and relationships?

0 = **None:** My anxiety doesn't affect my relationships.

1 = **Mild:** My anxiety slightly interferes with my relationships. Some of my friendships and other relationships have suffered, but, overall, my social life is still fulfilling.

2 = **Moderate:** I have experienced some interference with my social life, but I still have a few close relationships. I don't spend as much time with others as in the past, but I still socialize sometimes.

3 = **Severe:** My friendships and other relationships have suffered a lot because of anxiety. I do not enjoy social activities. I socialize very little.

4 = **Extreme:** My anxiety has completely disrupted my social activities. All of my relationships have suffered or ended. My family life is extremely strained.

Total Score: ____

Progress Record

ODSIS

| 20 |
| 18 |
| 16 |
| 14 |
| 12 |
| 10 |
| 8 |
| 6 |
| 4 |
| 2 |
| 0 |

Week 1 2 3 4 5 6 7 8 9 10 11 12 13 14 15 16 17 18 19 20 21 22 23 24 v

OASIS

| 20 |
| 18 |
| 16 |
| 14 |
| 12 |
| 10 |
| 8 |
| 6 |
| 4 |
| 2 |
| 0 |

Week 1 2 3 4 5 6 7 8 9 10 11 12 13 14 15 16 17 18 19 20 21 22 23 24 v

Other Assessment

| 20 |
| 18 |
| 16 |
| 14 |
| 12 |
| 10 |
| 8 |
| 6 |
| 4 |
| 2 |
| 0 |

Week 1 2 3 4 5 6 7 8 9 10 11 12 13 14 15 16 17 18 19 20 21 22 23 24 v

Worksheet 9.1: List of Emotional Behaviors

The purpose of this list is to identify emotional behaviors that you may use to avoid strong emotions, prevent emotions from becoming too intense, and/or reduce strong emotions once they have already begun. The list will help you later in treatment when you engage in emotion experiments, so that you can counter these unhelpful behaviors and ensure that the experiments are as effective as possible.

If you have trouble figuring out which columns to put a strategy in, that is OK. The most important part is that you begin to record the variety of emotion avoidance strategies you are engaging in currently.

Behavioral Avoidance	Cognitive Avoidance	Safety Signals

Worksheet 9.2: Alternative Action

Situation/Trigger	Emotion	Emotional Behavior	Alternative Action	Consequence of the Emotional Behavior vs. the Alternative Action

CHAPTER 10

Module 7: Experimenting with New Reactions to LGBTQ-Related Stress

Chapter 10 Overview

Many LGBTQ people falsely learn from an early age, based on their lived experience, that they do not have the right to stand up to stigma or to stand up for their needs or wants—and they continue to believe this even as they become adults. Today, you will learn how to recognize how you might be "silencing" yourself around others because you expect to experience stigma. In this session, you will also practice how to communicate your needs and wants, how to not hold yourself back, and how to be your most effective self in social situations.

Chapter 10 Outline

- Weekly Check-In
- Review Home Practice from Chapter 9
- How Does LGBTQ-Related Stress Impact Your Relationships?
- What Is Assertiveness?
- Becoming Assertive
- Saying "No"
- Assertiveness, Sex, and Substance Use
- Summary
- Home Practice: Assertiveness Practice

Take a minute to track your symptoms using the ODSIS and OASIS, located at the end of this chapter. You may also photocopy these forms or download multiple copies by searching for this book's title on the Oxford Academic platform at academic.oup.com. Do you notice any changes? What do you attribute these changes to?

Remember: Progress is not linear. Even as you approach the end of the treatment program, it's normal to see ups and downs in your symptoms. Sometimes, doing challenging things like countering emotional behaviors—like you did in the last chapter—can create some distress. The more you counter your emotional behaviors and engage in alternative behaviors that are aligned with your personal goals, the more you can expect your symptoms to ultimately decrease over time.

Review Home Practice from Chapter 9

Before we get started, take a look at Worksheet 9.1: List of Emotional Behaviors and Worksheet 9.2: Alternative Action. Remember, emotional behaviors are any behaviors that you use to (1) avoid feeling strong emotions, (2) prevent emotions from getting too intense, or (3) reduce strong emotions once they have already started.

How did you do with the worksheets?

- What emotional behaviors did you identify?
- Were you able to identify new behaviors to replace your emotional behaviors?
- Were you able to try out any of these new behaviors? What was that like?

It's sometimes hard to change emotional behaviors because this change involves facing the difficult emotions that come along with emotional behaviors. So, it's normal if this task was hard for you—nobody gets it just right on the first try!

Keep trying different new behaviors and track what works for you and how it feels. You can use the skills from the previous chapters to help you try new behaviors. For example:

1. *Challenge unhelpful thoughts.* If you think that you won't be able to cope with the emotions that a new behavior will bring on (e.g.,

discomfort, anxiety), try challenging this unhelpful thought and coming up with a more balanced thought (e.g., "I've done hard things before and gotten through them").

2. *Build motivation.* Motivation comes and goes. One way to keep your motivation high during these challenging activities is to go back to Chapter 4 in this workbook, where you weighed the pros and cons of changing versus staying the same. Think about all the reasons why these changes are important to you.

3. *Connect with the LGBTQ community.* Also keep in mind that new behaviors might focus on creating rewarding and enjoyable opportunities to form relationships with supportive members of the LGBTQ community.

How Does LGBTQ-Related Stress Impact Your Relationships?

Many LGBTQ people feel isolated, guilty, and ashamed because they live in a society that invalidates their experiences and denies them some of the same rights and respect that others get. You may have felt that you don't have the right to stand up to stigma, or that you should be ashamed of having needs in general. Many LGBTQ people expect rejection when expressing their needs. Although these tendencies might not feel directly connected to stigma happening right now, keep in mind that early experiences of stigma can impact LGBTQ people's behavior in ways that get learned, often outside of awareness, repeatedly over time.

For example:

Anders grew up getting messages that he was inferior because he was the only gay guy in his school. He didn't feel like he fit in with his cross-country team, especially when they talked about girls and dating. Anders learned to be quiet about his own desires and needs to avoid being rejected. Even now, he expects rejection and avoids talking about his personal life.

LGBTQ-related stress often results in uncomfortable feelings, thoughts of being inadequate or inferior, and, ultimately, difficulty communicating effectively and acting assertively. In this chapter you will learn about assertiveness and how you can use this skill to express your wants and needs with other people.

Think back to a time in your life when it was hard to stand up for your personal rights. For example, have you heard transphobic, biphobic, or homophobic comments but had difficulty speaking up and challenging them? Have you been in situations in which you couldn't come out or genuinely express yourself to others?

Like with other new behaviors, you can learn to be assertive. *Assertiveness* involves standing up for your needs and wants, while also respecting the needs of others. Box 10.1 shows how assertive behavior differs from passive and aggressive behavior.

Another way of thinking about assertiveness is "self-affirmation." In other words, you are affirming your own needs and wants by expressing them in situations with other people.

Maybe you're like Juan:

Juan's cousin always calls him late at night just to talk, but Juan has to get up early in the morning. The conversation is very one-sided, and Juan feels ignored and resents having to stay up late for this conversation.

What are some ways in which Juan could stand up for himself in this situation? Write down a few ideas here:

1. _____

2. _____

3. _____

Box 10.1. Spectrum of Interpersonal Behavior

PASSIVE   ASSERTIVE   AGGRESSIVE

Others' rights are respected.	Own *and* others' rights are respected.	Own rights are respected.
Own rights are denied.		Others' rights are denied.

Important Points About Assertiveness

By the end of this treatment, you will have skills to:

- Express yourself more freely and fully,
- Feel more confident and sure of yourself,
- Stand up for yourself in situations where you are treated unfairly, and
- Express your needs and wants to others.

It is important to understand a few things about assertiveness:

A Core Part of Assertiveness Is Identifying and Standing Up for Your Personal Rights

All people (including you) possess fundamental rights. These include the right to express your feelings, the right to make mistakes, and even the right to not assert yourself, among others. Take a moment and read aloud the "Assertiveness Bill of Rights," which appears in Box 10.2.

Consider the following questions as you read the Assertiveness Bill of Rights:

- Which of these rights do you sometimes forget that you have?
- What messages have you received as an LGBTQ person that may lead you to feel that you do not have these rights?
- What experiences have you had as an LGBTQ person that may make it difficult to assert these rights to other people?
- In what types of situations or with what types of people have you had the most difficulty asserting these rights?

LGBTQ-Related Stress Can Make LGBTQ People Forget That They Have These Rights

Because early and ongoing LGBTQ-related stress can teach LGBTQ people that they are inferior or should be rejected, it can stop them from being assertive. From the questions above, you may have started identifying how LGBTQ-related stress may interfere with your own assertive behavior.

How has past LGBTQ-related stress changed how you interact with others now? Ask yourself a few questions:

- What does society teach LGBTQ people about themselves?
- What stereotypes does society communicate about LGBTQ people?
- How might these stereotypes affect your assertive behavior or lack thereof?

Box 10.2. Assertiveness Bill of Rights

The following rights highlight the freedom you have to be yourself without disrespecting others.

The right to respect myself—who I am and what I do.

The right to have and express my own feelings and opinions appropriately and have them taken seriously by others—to make "I" statements about how I feel and think. For example, "I feel very uncomfortable with your decision."

The right to recognize my own needs as an individual—that is, separate from what is expected of me in particular roles such as "daughter," "brother," "partner," "student," or "worker."

The right to set my own priorities and ask for what I want rather than hoping someone will notice what I want.

The right to say "no" without feeling guilty.

The right to be treated with respect and not be taken for granted.

The right to offer no reasons or excuses for justifying my behaviors.

The right to make mistakes, recognizing that it is normal to make mistakes.

The right to ask for time to think something over. For example, when people ask me to do something, I have the right to say, "I would like to think it over and I will let you know my decision by the end of the week."

The right to say, "I don't know" and "I don't understand."

The right to change my mind.

The right to allow myself to enjoy my successes—that is, by being pleased with what I have done and sharing it with others.

The right to recognize that I am not responsible for the behavior of other adults.

The right to make my own decisions and deal with the consequences.

The right to respect other people and their right to be assertive and expect the same in return.

The right to choose *not* to assert myself.

Not Being Assertive Is a Type of Emotional Behavior

LGBTQ people may avoid being assertive because doing so would make them feel anxious, fearful of rejection, and/or self-conscious. Does this type of unassertiveness apply to you?

In the short term, avoiding these situations can work out, because you can avoid the difficult feelings that go along with them. However, in the long term, not being assertive can lead to depression, anxiety, hostility, relationship problems, and alcohol or drug abuse.

- What types of uncomfortable emotions do you avoid in the short term when you are unassertive?
- What are the long-term consequences to your life and goals of being unassertive?

Being Assertive Is Usually Better Than Being Passive

When people feel inadequate or afraid of rejection, they often engage in passive behaviors—accepting or allowing others to do whatever they want without questioning them or standing up to them. This might include avoiding uncomfortable discussions regarding sex, like requesting that your partner use a condom or discussing your sexual likes and dislikes.

Some people don't act assertively because they want to seem nice. And other people often like this! Others often get what they want, while the passive person doesn't. However, being passive all the time can lead to frustration or tension in relationships.

In contrast, being assertive involves identifying and standing up for your personal rights, even if someone else disagrees. Being assertive means communicating and behaving in a way that respects your own rights as well as the rights of other people.

Being assertive does not guarantee getting what you want or need, but the act of being assertive and choosing for yourself how to act usually results in a good feeling, regardless of whether the other person agrees with you, gives you what you asked for, or not.

- Think of a time when you were (or someone else was) assertive. How did this affect your relationship with that person (those people)? How did it affect the way you felt about yourself afterward?

Being Assertive Is Not the Same as Being Aggressive or Passive-Aggressive

When people feel inadequate or afraid of rejection, they sometimes also act aggressively—getting what they want by threatening, yelling, or engaging in physical violence.

You may have also heard of passive-aggressiveness. Passive-aggressive people repeatedly push away their own wants—they go along with what other people want rather than what they themselves want (i.e., the passive part).

But then they respond negatively (i.e., the aggressive part) to these actions on the part of others. Aggression and passive-aggression are both emotional behaviors that can introduce more conflict into relationships. In contrast, being assertive can build trust and openness in relationships over time.

- Can you think of a time when you (or someone else) were either aggressive or passive-aggressive?
- How did this affect the relationship?
- How did it affect the way you felt about yourself afterward?

Putting It All Together

The assertiveness skills you'll learn today combat all of these behaviors by helping you express your rights, needs, or goals in a *calm, confident, and positive way*. This may include things like saying "no" to an unreasonable request, or appropriately asking someone to stop doing something that is bothersome or even hurtful. By being appropriately assertive, people often develop self-respect and also earn the respect of others.

Becoming Assertive

You can increase your ability to be assertive through the following three steps:

1. Identify a challenging situation in your life in which it is hard to assert your needs and wants.
2. Challenge your unassertive thoughts.
3. Act appropriately assertively.

Let's go through each of these steps in detail.

Step 1: Identify a Challenging Situation

To complete this first step, fill out Worksheet 10.1: Asserting Yourself in Challenging Situations, which is located at the end of this chapter and also available for download by searching for this book's title on the Oxford Academic platform at academic.oup.com. Be sure to choose safe situations in which to assertive yourself. There are likely many safe situations in which you can assert yourself. Examples of unsafe situations might be those that might reasonably put you at risk for psychological harm (e.g., verbal abuse) as well as other serious negative consequences (e.g., being kicked out of your home, being financially cut-off, losing your job or a scholarship) if you were to assert yourself. Also be sure to assess your physical safety in situations in which you practice assertiveness.

Do not practice this skill in situations that have the potential for physical harm. For example, it is important to practice this skill with people in your life who do not have a history of or tendency toward violence.

Step 2: Challenge Unassertive Thoughts

How you think about yourself and your personal rights will influence whether you choose to be assertive. Fears of being judged, criticized, and even harassed or attacked can negatively impact your ability to behave assertively. Some negative feelings and thoughts in these situations are perfectly reasonable, while many are probably not helpful.

Earlier, when you learned about automatic thoughts, you learned to think more flexibly. That new flexibility is also helpful here as you assertively face situations that you might have avoided before.

Go back to the situation that you identified in Step 1 (in Worksheet 10.1). To challenge unassertive thoughts, try to identify the automatic thoughts you had in that situation and think of new interpretations. To do that, answer the questions listed on Worksheet 10.2: Building Assertive Thoughts, located at the end of this chapter. You may also download a copy of the worksheet by searching for this book's title on the Oxford Academic platform at academic.oup.com.

Here's an example that many people who have faced unassertiveness can relate to: Say your friend Katja always borrows money without repaying it. You might *think* that if you stand up for yourself, she will think that you are a rude, awful person and your friendship will be ruined. So, you don't ask for your money back and, instead, simmer with anger about how unfair she is being.

The problem is that these angry thoughts you're having could start to negatively affect your friendship. You might start interacting with her differently, possibly in a subtly more hostile way, or start complaining about her to other friends. But if you instead *think* that you have the right to get your money back and ask her in a polite way, Katja may respect your decision to be upfront with her. Also, you may no longer have negative thoughts about her.

This example shows how your *thoughts* can impact the way that you eventually *behave*.

Instead, you could replace these thoughts with other more helpful and balanced thoughts. For example, "If Katja does get offended, it's not the end of the world. She might even respect me being direct with her. I have a right to get my money back. The results of my actions will probably not be as terrible as I *think*."

Step 3: Act Assertively

Now, let's return to the situation you identified in Step 1 (Worksheet 10.1) again. Practice saying aloud what you might say in that situation. Yes, you should actually say this stuff aloud! Why? It might sound weird, but there's a good reason to say it aloud: The more realistic your practice, the more likely it will be to help you make it happen in real life. If you're working with a therapist, you might also do this in a roleplay with your therapist.

While you're saying it aloud, pay attention to your posture, eye contact, and volume. Make eye contact. Assume a confident posture. Speak loudly and without mumbling. Express your thoughts and feelings as clearly and honestly as possible. You don't have to apologize for stating your wants and needs. You can even record yourself on your phone to see how assertive your behavior is from an "outsider's" perspective.

Now that you've said this aloud, fill out Worksheet 10.3: Reflecting on Acting Assertively to see how it went. This worksheet is located at the end of this chapter and is also available for download by searching for this book's title on the Oxford Academic platform at academic.oup.com.

Saying "No"

Many people find that "no" seems to be one of the hardest words to say—even when a request is unreasonable. Do you find it hard to say "no" to other people? This is one example of unassertive behavior. Saying "no" can be both important and helpful. If you don't say this one simple word, you might be drawn into situations that you don't want to be in.

There are many reasons why people have a hard time saying "no" or refusing requests from others. For example, you may not want to be seen as mean and selfish. Or, you may not want to be rejected by others, so you go along with what they want. But as discussed above, not asserting yourself can start to negatively impact your relationships, as you can start feeling angry or resentful over time.

If you have problems saying "no," try to practice it:

1. Be direct and honest so that you can make your point effectively.
2. If you are finding it difficult to say "no," you can tell the person that you are finding it difficult.
3. You don't need to apologize and give lots of reasons for saying "no." It's your right to say "no" if you don't want to do something (this is in Box 10.2, Assertiveness Bill of Rights).

4. Remember that it's better in the long run to be truthful than to grow bitter and resentful, or to act passive-aggressively.

Assertiveness, Sex, and Substance Use

Not being assertive can cause serious problems for LGBTQ people's mental health. Many LGBTQ folks report that feeling worthless or having low self-esteem gets in the way of engaging in healthy activities and relationships. For instance, in some cases they may cope with their negative emotions in these contexts with emotional behaviors, including alcohol and substance use.

DeShawn is a bisexual man who drinks alcohol and sometimes uses other drugs when he goes to a bar to gather the courage to talk to an attractive person. When having sex, DeShawn does not believe that he has the right to ask that they use condoms or to discuss sexual health. He worries that if he does ask these questions, he might turn off his potential partner. In this situation, DeShawn thinks, *"Who am I to ask this attractive person about their sexual health?"* *"If I insist on using a condom, they will reject me, and think I am sick"* and *"It's easier for now to just go without a condom."*

If both DeShawn and his partner have been using substances, their ability to make decisions and to assertively discuss their sexual health may be impaired, which only adds to DeShawn's difficulty asserting himself. In the short term, DeShawn may make a decision that allows him to avoid his uncomfortable emotions, but this decision could also have long-term effects, like eroding his ability to assert himself in future situations or acquiring a sexually transmitted infection.

Think about your own life. Have there have been times where, like DeShawn, you didn't know how to say "no"?

In romantic relationships, being assertive is also important and can affect, for example, agreements regarding sex with outside partners or the decision to use alcohol or other substances together.

By recognizing that LGBTQ-related stress is sometimes the source of these difficulties in relationships, you can become motivated to stand up to this stress. As a result, you can make better decisions that support your health.

Summary

In this chapter you learned about how LGBTQ-related stress can affect your ability to stand up to stigma and express your needs and wants.

You thought about the ways in which you might silence yourself around others because you expect to be rejected or mistreated. You learned about your personal rights and being assertive. You also learned how to assess your own level of assertiveness, how to challenge unassertive thoughts, and how to be assertive in your life. Finally, you learned why it's important to be able to say "no," and how sexual health and substance use decisions are tied to being assertive.

With some practice, you will build the skills of expressing your own needs and wants in a clear and effective way. Being assertive is a skill that can be learned—you can do it!

Home Practice: Assertiveness Practice

Now that you are at the end of this chapter, you're ready to put what you've learned about assertiveness into practice!

Practice being assertive *three times* over the next week. Record your progress on Worksheets 10.4 to 10.6: Record of Assertiveness Practice, located at the end of this chapter.

There are three separate worksheets so that you can record all three assertive practice exercises. You may also download these worksheets by searching for this book's title on the Oxford Academic platform at academic.oup.com. Challenge yourself to find increasingly difficult situations that will be helpful to your progress.

Try thinking of three situations that are likely to come up in the next week in which you could practice assertive behavior (alternatively, you could try being assertive in the same situation multiple times this week):

1. _____

2. _____

3. _____

As with all the other home practice activities, remember to think of this as "practice"—just like with sports, school, or hobbies, practice leads to getting better. If you get frustrated, that's OK—practice can be hard! Feel free to take a break. It can help to try out different times to work on the exercises until you find the time that works for you.

Remember: Regular practice is more important than doing it "perfectly."

Overall Depression Severity and Interference Scale (ODSIS)

Instructions: The following items ask about depression. For each item, indicate the number for the answer that best describes your experience over the past week.

—1. In the past week, how often have you felt depressed?

    0 = **No depression** in the past week.

    1 = **Infrequent depression**. Felt depressed a few times.

    2 = **Occasional depression**. Felt depressed as much of the time as not.

    3 = **Frequent depression**. Felt depressed most of the time.

    4 = **Constant depression**. Felt depressed all of the time.

—2. In the past week, when you have felt depressed, how intense or severe was your depression?

    0 = **Little or None**: Depression was absent or barely noticeable.

    1 = **Mild**: Depression was at a low level.

    2 = **Moderate**: Depression was intense at times.

    3 = **Severe**: Depression was intense much of the time.

    4 = **Extreme**: Depression was overwhelming.

—3. In the past week, how often did you have difficulty engaging in or being interested in activities you normally enjoy because of depression?

    0 = **None**: I had no difficulty engaging in or being interested in activities that I normally enjoy because of depression.

    1 = **Infrequent**: A few times I had difficulty engaging in or being interested in activities that I normally enjoy because of depression. My lifestyle was not affected.

    2 = **Occasional**: I had some difficulty engaging in or being interested in activities that I normally enjoy because of depression. My lifestyle has only changed in minor ways.

    3 = **Frequent**: I have considerable difficulty engaging in or being interested in activities that I normally enjoy because of depression. I have made significant changes in my lifestyle because of being unable to become interested in activities I used to enjoy.

    4 = **All the Time**: I have been unable to participate in or be interested in activities that I normally enjoy because of depression. My lifestyle has been extensively affected and I no longer do things that I used to enjoy.

—4. In the past week, how much did your depression interfere with your ability to do the things you needed to do at work, at school, or at home?

    0 = **None**: No interference at work/home/school from depression.

    1 = **Mild**: My depression has caused some interference at work/home/school. Things are more difficult, but everything that needs to be done is still getting done.

    2 = **Moderate**: My depression definitely interferes with tasks. Most things are still getting done, but few things are being done as well as in the past.

    3 = **Severe**: My depression has really changed my ability to get things done. Some tasks are still being done, but many things are not. My performance has definitely suffered.

4 = **Extreme**: My depression has become incapacitating. I am unable to complete tasks and have had to leave school, have quit or been fired from my job, or have been unable to complete tasks at home and have faced consequences like bill collectors, eviction, etc.

—5. In the past week, how much has depression interfered with your social life and relationships?

0 = **None**: My depression doesn't affect my relationships.

1 = **Mild**: My depression slightly interferes with my relationships. Some of my friendships and other relationships have suffered, but, overall, my social life is still fulfilling.

2 = **Moderate**: I have experienced some interference with my social life, but I still have a few close relationships. I don't spend as much time with others as in the past, but I still socialize sometimes.

3 = **Severe**: My friendships and other relationships have suffered a lot because of depression. I do not enjoy social activities. I socialize very little.

4 = **Extreme**: My depression has completely disrupted my social activities. All of my relationships have suffered or ended. My family life is extremely strained.

Total Score: ____

Overall Anxiety Severity and Interference Scale (OASIS)

Instructions: The following items ask about anxiety and fear. For each item, indicate the number for the answer that best describes your experience over the past week.

—1. In the past week, how often have you felt anxious?

0 = **No anxiety** in the past week.

1 = **Infrequent anxiety.** Felt anxious a few times.

2 = **Occasional anxiety.** Felt anxious as much of the time as not. It was hard to relax.

3 = **Frequent anxiety.** Felt anxious most of the time. It was very difficult to relax.

4 = **Constant anxiety.** Felt anxious all of the time and never really relaxed.

—2. In the past week, when you have felt anxious, how intense or severe was your anxiety?

0 = **Little or None:** Anxiety was absent or barely noticeable.

1 = **Mild:** Anxiety was at a low level. It was possible to relax when I tried. Physical symptoms were only slightly uncomfortable.

2 = **Moderate:** Anxiety was distressing at times. It was hard to relax or concentrate, but I could do it if I tried. Physical symptoms were uncomfortable.

3 = **Severe:** Anxiety was intense much of the time. It was very difficult to relax or focus on anything else. Physical symptoms were extremely uncomfortable.

4 = **Extreme:** Anxiety was overwhelming. It was impossible to relax at all. Physical symptoms were unbearable.

—3. In the past week, how often did you avoid situations, places, objects, or activities because of anxiety or fear?

0 = **None:** I do not avoid places, situations, activities, or things because of fear.

1 = **Infrequent:** I avoid something once in a while, but will usually face the situation or confront the object. My lifestyle is not affected.

2 = **Occasional:** I have some fear of certain situations, places, or objects, but it is still manageable. My lifestyle has only changed in minor ways. I always or almost always avoid the things I fear when I'm alone, but can handle them if someone comes with me.

3 = **Frequent:** I have considerable fear and really try to avoid the things that frighten me. I have made significant changes in my lifestyle to avoid the object, situation, activity, or place.

4 = **All the Time:** Avoiding objects, situations, activities, or places has taken over my life. My lifestyle has been extensively affected and I no longer do things that I used to enjoy.

—4. In the past week, how much did your anxiety interfere with your ability to do the things you needed to do at work, at school, or at home?

0 = **None:** No interference at work/home/school from anxiety.

1 = **Mild:** My anxiety has caused some interference at work/home/school. Things are more difficult, but everything that needs to be done is still getting done.

2 = **Moderate:** My anxiety definitely interferes with tasks. Most things are still getting done, but few things are being done as well as in the past.

3 = **Severe:** My anxiety has really changed my ability to get things done. Some tasks are still being done, but many things are not. My performance has definitely suffered.

4 = **Extreme:** My anxiety has become incapacitating. I am unable to complete tasks and have had to leave school, have quit or been fired from my job, or have been unable to complete tasks at home and have faced consequences like bill collectors, eviction, etc.

—5. In the past week, how much has anxiety interfered with your social life and relationships?

0 = **None:** My anxiety doesn't affect my relationships.

1 = **Mild:** My anxiety slightly interferes with my relationships. Some of my friendships and other relationships have suffered, but, overall, my social life is still fulfilling.

2 = **Moderate:** I have experienced some interference with my social life, but I still have a few close relationships. I don't spend as much time with others as in the past, but I still socialize sometimes.

3 = **Severe:** My friendships and other relationships have suffered a lot because of anxiety. I do not enjoy social activities. I socialize very little.

4 = **Extreme:** My anxiety has completely disrupted my social activities. All of my relationships have suffered or ended. My family life is extremely strained.

Total Score: ___

ODSIS

```
20 ─────────────────────────────────────────
18 ─────────────────────────────────────────
16 ─────────────────────────────────────────
14 ─────────────────────────────────────────
12 ─────────────────────────────────────────
10 ─────────────────────────────────────────
 8 ─────────────────────────────────────────
 6 ─────────────────────────────────────────
 4 ─────────────────────────────────────────
 2 ─────────────────────────────────────────
 0 ─────────────────────────────────────────
```

| Week 1 | 2 | 3 | 4 | 5 | 6 | 7 | 8 | 9 | 10 | 11 | 12 | 13 | 14 | 15 | 16 | 17 | 18 | 19 | 20 | 21 | 22 | 23 | 24 | v |

OASIS

```
20 ─────────────────────────────────────────
18 ─────────────────────────────────────────
16 ─────────────────────────────────────────
14 ─────────────────────────────────────────
12 ─────────────────────────────────────────
10 ─────────────────────────────────────────
 8 ─────────────────────────────────────────
 6 ─────────────────────────────────────────
 4 ─────────────────────────────────────────
 2 ─────────────────────────────────────────
 0 ─────────────────────────────────────────
```

| Week 1 | 2 | 3 | 4 | 5 | 6 | 7 | 8 | 9 | 10 | 11 | 12 | 13 | 14 | 15 | 16 | 17 | 18 | 19 | 20 | 21 | 22 | 23 | 24 | v |

Other Assessment

```
20 ─────────────────────────────────────────
18 ─────────────────────────────────────────
16 ─────────────────────────────────────────
14 ─────────────────────────────────────────
12 ─────────────────────────────────────────
10 ─────────────────────────────────────────
 8 ─────────────────────────────────────────
 6 ─────────────────────────────────────────
 4 ─────────────────────────────────────────
 2 ─────────────────────────────────────────
 0 ─────────────────────────────────────────
```

| Week 1 | 2 | 3 | 4 | 5 | 6 | 7 | 8 | 9 | 10 | 11 | 12 | 13 | 14 | 15 | 16 | 17 | 18 | 19 | 20 | 21 | 22 | 23 | 24 | v |

Worksheet 10.1: Asserting Yourself in Challenging Situations

Consider a situation in which you may currently be denying your personal rights as an individual and as an LGBTQ person. Write it here. (Remember, you always have the right to express your thoughts and feelings, even if others may not always agree with them.)

Using the situation that you just identified above, write your answers to the following questions below. What rights do you have in this situation? (Hint: you can go back to the Assertiveness Bill of Rights.)

What makes it hard to stand up for your rights in this situation? Think about your experiences of LGBTQ-related stress.

How would you usually respond in this type of situation?

Think about the other person or people involved in this situation. What would you like to say to this person?

How would you like this person to respond?

What could you say or what actions could you take to achieve your goals?

Worksheet 10.2: Building Assertive Thoughts

Looking at the situation you described in Worksheet 10.1, what goes on in your head when you imagine yourself in this situation?
Do you need approval from others?
Is the thought 100% true?
Is the result you fear definitely going to happen?
What do you know that says it may not happen?
Even if it did happen, is it the end of the world? Could you handle it?
Does it make you a bad or worthless person if it does happen?

Worksheet 10.3: Reflecting on Acting Assertively

What did you like about the Acting Assertively exercise? What didn't you like?

What thoughts, feelings, and behaviors did you notice before and during the exercise?

If you had negative automatic thoughts, like "this isn't going to work" or "I can't do this," how might you change your automatic thoughts?

What do you think you need to keep practicing?

Worksheet 10.4: Record of Assertiveness Practice (Exercise 1)

Identify situations in which you want to be more assertive in the upcoming week, and write down your reactions.

Assertiveness Experiment:

_____

_____

_____

Prior to the assertiveness experiment:

Anticipatory Distress (0–8): _____

Thoughts, Behaviors, and Bodily Feelings you noticed before the experiment:

_____

_____

_____

Re-evaluate your automatic appraisals about the experiment:

_____

_____

_____

After completing the assertiveness experiment:

Thoughts, Behaviors, and Bodily Feelings you noticed during the experiment:

_____

_____

_____

Maximum distress during the experiment (0–8): _____

Distress at the end of the experiment (0–8): _____

Any attempts to avoid your emotions (distraction, safety signals, etc.)?

_____

_____

_____

What did you take away from this assertiveness experiment? Did your feared outcomes occur? If so, how were you able to cope with them?

_____

_____

_____

Worksheet 10.5: Record of Assertiveness Practice (Exercise 2)

Identify situations in which you want to be more assertive in the upcoming week and write down your reactions.

Assertiveness Experiment:

_____

_____

_____

<u>Prior to the assertiveness experiment:</u>

Anticipatory Distress (0–8): _____

Thoughts, Behaviors, and Bodily Feelings you noticed before the experiment:

_____

_____

_____

Re-evaluate your automatic appraisals about the experiment:

_____

_____

_____

<u>After completing the assertiveness experiment:</u>

Thoughts, Behaviors, and Bodily Feelings you noticed during the experiment:

_____

_____

_____

Maximum distress during the experiment (0–8): _____

Distress at the end of the experiment (0–8): _____

Any attempts to avoid your emotions (distraction, safety signals, etc.)?

_____

_____

_____

What did you take away from this assertiveness experiment? Did your feared outcomes occur? If so, how were you able to cope with them?

_____

_____

_____

Worksheet 10.6: Record of Assertiveness Practice (Exercise 3)

Identify situations in which you want to be more assertive in the upcoming week and write down your reactions.

Assertiveness Experiment:

_____

_____

_____

Prior to the assertiveness experiment:

Anticipatory Distress (0–8): _____

Thoughts, Behaviors, and Bodily Feelings you noticed before the experiment:

_____

_____

_____

Re-evaluate your automatic appraisals about the experiment:

_____

_____

_____

After completing the assertiveness experiment:

Thoughts, Behaviors, and Bodily Feelings you noticed during the experiment:

_____

_____

_____

Maximum distress during the experiment (0–8): _____

Distress at the end of the experiment (0–8): _____

Any attempts to avoid your emotions (distraction, safety signals, etc.)?

_____

_____

_____

What did you take away from this assertiveness experiment? Did your feared outcomes occur? If so, how were you able to cope with them?

_____

_____

_____

Module 8: Emotion Exposures for Countering LGBTQ-Related Stress

Chapter 11 Overview

The skills you have been learning in this treatment program aren't meant to stay in your head: The best way to test out your negative beliefs about your emotions—and the situations that cause them—is to face them. By confronting emotional situations with the skills you've learned so far, you can learn to manage any strong emotions. In this chapter, you will learn how "emotion exposures" allow you to approach situations and feelings that you usually avoid. As you will see in this chapter, emotion exposures are helpful for several reasons and give you the chance to put your new skills into practice.

Chapter 11 Outline

- Weekly Check-In
- Review Home Practice from Chapter 10
- LGBTQ-Related Stress and Avoidance
- Avoiding Unpleasant Bodily Feelings
- Avoiding Unpleasant Situations
- Designing Effective Emotion Exposures for *You*
- Summary
- Home Practice 1: Emotion Exposures to Cause Unpleasant Bodily Feelings

- Home Practice 2: Emotion Exposures to Approach Uncomfortable Situations
- Key Things to Remember About Emotion Exposures

Weekly Check-In

Take a minute to track your symptoms using the ODSIS and OASIS, located at the end of this chapter. You may also photocopy these forms or download multiple copies by searching for this book's title on the Oxford Academic platform at academic.oup.com. Do you notice any changes? What do you attribute these changes to?

Review Home Practice from Chapter 10

Identify a situation in which you practiced being assertive. What did you think, feel, and do while you practiced being assertive?

_____

_____

_____

_____

Then, using Worksheet 11.1: Reviewing Your Progress, reflect upon your work to maintain the skills you learned in earlier chapters. The worksheet is located at the end of this chapter and is also available for download by searching for this book's title on the Oxford Academic platform at academic.oup.com.

LGBTQ-Related Stress and Avoidance

LGBTQ-related stress often leads LGBTQ people to feel strong negative emotions. Because LGBTQ people have these emotional experiences frequently, they can often lead to emotional behaviors like avoiding close relationships, avoiding being vulnerable, or avoiding situations that produce uncomfortable feelings. By approaching these experiences using the skills discussed here, LGBTQ people can develop healthier responses to LGBTQ-related stress. Let's take some examples:

Dishon avoids going places where other gay men will be present. He is afraid they won't be welcoming and that he won't have anything to talk to them about. Dishon has a goal of making more gay male friends, but is not sure where to start.

Rula never had friends growing up. She formed her first real friendship in college with a woman named Lisa, but this friendship ended poorly when Rula developed feelings for Lisa. One night, Rula attempted to kiss Lisa while drunk. Lisa pushed Rula away and began to slowly distance herself from Rula, and Rula was devastated. She had finally found a friend, and now she had ruined the friendship. After this, Rula did all she could to avoid being rejected again. Her friendships were focused mostly on having a good time, drinking on the weekends, and smoking pot. She kept people at a distance to protect herself from getting hurt later on.

Perhaps you see yourself in Dave or Rula. Or maybe you don't exactly relate to people like they do, but there are some situations that you avoid and you suspect this avoidance has its roots in LGBTQ-related stress.

Before we get to the actual situations that you avoid, let's first look at why these situations *feel* so scary for you.

Avoiding Unpleasant Bodily Feelings

Imagine yourself in Diana's shoes:

Diana has had several panic attacks in her life where her heart beat so fast she thought it would beat out of her chest. Her breath was so short she felt like she might pass out. Now anytime Diana has a fast heart rate, she interprets it as a sign that a full-blown panic attack is around the corner.

Or maybe you're like Pegah:

Pegah gets nervous in social situations, feeling hot and sweaty anytime they have to interact with others. Now anytime they get hot and sweaty, they are afraid that other people can see they're anxious and will judge them for it.

When faced with uncomfortable situations, some people experience other bodily feelings like knots in their stomach, cramping, or nausea. Like

Diana and Pegah, these feelings might cause intense fear, which often leads people to avoid the situations that caused them.

Their avoidance is understandable but probably isn't helpful most of the time. For example, because Diana was upset by panic attacks she had had in the past, she was scared of getting them again. When she was panicking, she wasn't able to function and had a difficult time breathing. So Diana did what most people would do: She avoided anything that would cause a feeling that was at all similar to her panic attacks. This worked for a while, until she began having problems at work.

When she felt the pressure of a deadline or stressful project, she experienced tension in her chest, a symptom she felt when a panic attack was about to occur. Because of this chest tension, Diana believed that something bad was going to occur—like a panic attack—and this stopped her from moving forward with the project at hand. As a result, she started missing deadlines on important projects at work. Diana's intense bodily feelings made her *feel* like something bad was about to occur. But this is not true in most cases.

Given this, it's no surprise that these bodily feelings contribute to the urge to avoid emotions. It's totally normal if your first inclination is to avoid painful emotions, but remember that trying to escape from strong emotions tends to backfire in the long run. That's what happens with bodily feelings too. If you try to avoid having certain bodily feelings (or being in the situations that have caused these feelings), they will seem more overwhelming over time. Again, this is because avoiding something teaches you that you can't cope with it.

When, where, and how our bodily feelings occur is very important in figuring out how to interpret them. Let's consider the example of children having fun on a playground. When a child goes down a slide, their stomach might drop, and they might feel lightheaded when they land at the bottom. The whole purpose of merry-go-rounds on playgrounds is to make kids dizzy—so dizzy they can't stand up when they get off. Playing tag can bring on a racing heart, sweatiness, and shortness of breath—all from running around. When these bodily feelings happen to a child on the playground, they are considered *good* feelings—something kids purposely bring on!

But consider this: These are the very *same* feelings that can seem so scary and threatening in a different situation—for example, as an adult, giving a speech or entering a situation that scares them.

This means that the bodily feelings themselves are not the problem—instead, it is your *interpretation* of these feelings that makes them so scary and uncomfortable. By themselves, bodily feelings don't *have* to be bad or threatening. As we mentioned, bodily feelings are a normal, integral part of emotions. It is your *interpretation* of bodily feelings that makes them feel bad. Let's break this down to see how this applies to you.

Note that "panic attacks" come from what we consider a "fear of fear" cycle. That is, a symptom of anxiety comes on for whatever reason. The person then has anxiety about the fact that this symptom is happening. For example, they think, "Oh my gosh, my heart is beating too fast, I must be having a heart attack," or "Oh no, I am feeling a little nauseous—I am going to throw up uncontrollably." Having these anxiety-provoking thoughts in reaction to the physical symptoms actually makes the anxiety symptoms worse. And then the symptoms getting worse makes the thoughts happen more, and the anxiety keeps escalating into a full-blown panic attack.

The good news is that your interpretation of your bodily feelings is something that can be changed. In fact, you can actually become more comfortable with these feelings over time. We will help you achieve this by using exercises designed to bring on the same bodily feelings that come up when you have strong emotions. We will ask you to practice experiencing these feelings again and again, without doing anything to make them go away. We do this for several reasons:

1. By doing these exercises, you can experience what a physical feeling feels like on its own, separate from any interpretation of what it might mean. When people explore these feelings without judgment—while focusing on what they're actually feeling in the present moment (versus what they might feel in the future)—the feelings don't seem as bad.
2. By repeatedly causing these feelings, you will learn that you can cope with them, even when you don't do anything to manage them.
3. Finally, the more you practice feeling these feelings, the more you will get used to them. They might start to feel routine to you—even boring!

The idea is that when these bodily feelings come along with a strong emotion in the real world, you will know that these feelings are safe and manageable, even if they are uncomfortable. Having bodily feelings come up during an emotional experience will no longer make your emotions feel hard to handle.

Avoiding Unpleasant Situations

So far, we have talked about avoiding unpleasant feelings, but avoiding feelings may not be such a problem for you. Instead, you might avoid unpleasant *situations*, like:

- difficult conversations with loved ones or coworkers,
- hanging out with cisgender or heterosexual people,
- making friends within the LGBTQ community,
- having sex without using substances,
- expressing affection towards romantic partners, or
- being vulnerable.

Take Miguel as an example:

Miguel is a gay trans man who avoids dating and even gets anxious when another man talks to him. Although he wants to be in a relationship, he can't bring himself to take the steps necessary to be in a relationship. Miguel is not avoiding his bodily feelings; rather, he is avoiding dating and talking to potential romantic partners.

To help with this, Miguel and his therapist decided to do an activity together:

Miguel and a guy at his gym have glanced at each other a few times while working out. Miguel isn't sure if the guy is interested, but Miguel would really like to talk to him. Before Miguel's next therapy session, he and his therapist agreed that Miguel would start a conversation with this guy. The idea of this conversation makes Miguel's heart race and his mind go blank. Miguel's therapist reminds him that it's not about making that fear and anxiety go away. Rather, it's about noticing the fear and anxiety and *sticking to his goal* of meeting men.

We've talked about two types of avoidance so far: avoiding unpleasant bodily feelings (including symptoms of anxiety) and avoiding unpleasant situations.

- Which of the two do you find yourself avoiding the most?
- Do you find yourself avoiding uncomfortable bodily feelings? Does the slightest twinge of tension, nausea, or dizziness cause unnecessary fear?
- Or are there specific situations you avoid that cause you problems? Do you feel lonely, but can't seem to get yourself to attend social events where you could meet new friends or romantic partners?
- Or perhaps you avoid both unpleasant feelings and situations.

Choose the type of avoidance that is most relevant to you. You can choose both types of avoidance if that applies to you:

- Bodily feelings
- Unpleasant situations

Now it's time to try to break these avoidance patterns down so that you can get used to your unpleasant emotions and see that you can cope. Emotion exposures are exercises that are specifically designed (by you) to cause the strong emotional responses you usually avoid. From previous sessions, you know all the skills for how to respond to these emotions. Now it's time for the final piece: stepping outside your comfort zone!

These exposures will help you to learn a few things:

1. Any uncomfortable emotions you feel are temporary. Even without changing your behavior or situation, your negative emotions will eventually fade or go away.
2. You can cope with negative emotions better than you think.
3. You can do things that are important to you even when your emotions are intense.
4. Your interpretation of bodily feelings can be changed. You can become more comfortable with these feelings over time.

Let's look at some of the bodily feelings and situations that you avoid by using Worksheet 11.2: Emotion Exposure Ladder, which is located at the end of this chapter and also available for download by searching for this book's title on the Oxford Academic platform at academic.oup.com.

Think of this worksheet as a ladder, with bodily feelings or situations that cause the most uncomfortable emotions at the top, and those that cause the least uncomfortable emotions at the bottom. Sometimes it can be helpful to start at the bottom, with the less challenging situations, and then work your way up to the more challenging situations. Rate how much you avoid each of the situations you describe and how upset (or distressed) each situation makes you from 0 to 8 (where 8 is the highest).

To help you, Miguel's Completed Emotion Exposure Ladder, which he completed with his therapist, is shown in Figure 11.1 (on p. 213). You can see that all of his ladder items are focused on his ultimate goal of being in a romantic relationship. You can also see that Miguel focused on situational avoidance, rather than avoidance of bodily feelings, but the general principles in creating the ladder are the same for both—put the most uncomfortable bodily feelings or situations on the top and the least uncomfortable bodily feelings or situations on the bottom.

Now it's your turn! Fill in Worksheet 11.2: Emotion Exposure Ladder, which is located at the end of this chapter and also available for download by searching for this book's title on the Oxford Academic platform at academic.oup.com.

Note: For ideas on how to complete the worksheet, check out the lists of exercises in Home Practice 1 ("Emotion Exposures to Cause Unpleasant Bodily Feelings") and Home Practice 2 ("Emotion Exposures to Approach Uncomfortable Situations"). Choose the exercises that are most relevant to you and add them to your Emotion Exposure Ladder or create your own.

Remember these tips when building your Emotion Exposure Ladder:

- **Try to plan emotion exposures in a variety of different situations** (e.g., home, school, in public, alone). This can help the lessons you learn about coping with emotions really stick.
- **Try combining more than one emotion exposure in the same task**. Once you get used to doing some of your exposures, consider combining them. For example, if feeling jittery and talking to straight people both make you anxious, you might include "drink a large cup of coffee, then talk to my straight coworker."

- **Make the Emotion Exposure Ladder your own.** You can make your Emotion Exposure Ladder longer than eight items or create a new Emotion Exposure Ladder after you complete the tasks on the first one.

Summary

Sometimes, people may feel inclined to avoid physical sensations that are typically associated with stressful situations, such as increased heart rate, sweaty palms, and lightheadedness. Other people might avoid unpleasant situations or emotions. Unfortunately, attempts to avoid these physical sensations, unpleasant situations, or uncomfortable emotions can make them seem even more threatening and distressing. The best way to test out your negative beliefs about your emotions (and the situations that cause them) is to face them and see what happens. You can do this at your own pace, one step at a time.

Home Practice 1: Emotion Exposures to Cause Unpleasant Bodily Feelings

Some people fear bodily sensations or physical symptoms of anxiety. Just like other types of anxiety, the best way to combat this fear is by exposing yourself to the thing you fear. So, in this case, it means exposing yourself to physical symptoms that you normally would be afraid of having. It means actually bringing on these symptoms on purpose, in order to be able to emotionally relearn that they are not dangerous. Here are some more details of what to do.

In order to do these exercises, you will need a stopwatch or timer as well as a thin straw (or coffee stirrer) for exercise #2.

Review Worksheet 11.3: Bodily Feelings Exposure Test, located near the end of this chapter, and try each of the exercises listed there (and explained below) for 60 seconds without stopping. These exercises, such as breathing through a thin straw, spinning in a swivel chair, and running in place, are intended to bring on bodily feelings that can be unpleasant when they occur as part of depression or anxiety symptoms. After engaging in these exercises each for 60 seconds, be sure to record the bodily feelings you experience and how distressed you feel on a 0-to-8 scale (0 = no distress, 8 = extreme distress). Finally, rate how similar these bodily feelings are to the feelings you have when you are experiencing strong emotions on a scale of 0 to 8 (0 = not at all similar to my emotion, 8 = extremely similar). Worksheet 11.3 is also available for download by searching for this book's title on the Oxford Academic platform at academic.oup.com.

Wait until the bodily feelings have mostly gone away before attempting the next exercise. Remember to do the bodily feeling exposure exercises so that you feel your bodily feelings as strongly as possible. You may only be able to engage in the exercises for a short period of time at first.

Remember to not stop the exposure until you've fully felt your feelings. This is because ending the exposure upon first noticing the bodily feelings will reinforce your fear of those bodily feelings.

Here are the exercises:

1. **Hyperventilation:** Take rapid, deep breaths through your mouth, using a lot of force, as if you were blowing up a balloon really fast. This exercise is likely to cause you to feel lightheaded, dizzy, or like things around you aren't real.
2. **Breathe through a thin straw:** Breathe through a thin straw or coffee stirrer while blocking air from your nose. Make sure that you're only taking in air through the straw, without breathing around it. This exercise will make it feel like you can't get enough air, even though you can, and it is designed to make you feel anxious. You will get the most benefit from it if you stick with it for the full minute.
3. **Spin in circles:** Stand up and turn around quickly (approximately one full rotation every three seconds). You can do this with your eyes open or closed. Alternatively, you can spin in a chair that swivels. If you do this exercise standing, consider doing it near a chair or couch where you can sit down afterwards. This exercise is designed to make you feel dizzy, lightheaded, and disoriented.
4. **Run in place:** Run in place while lifting your knees as high as you can. This exercise is designed to cause rapid heart rate, shortness of breath, flushed cheeks, and increased body heat.

While you're completing these exercises:

- Notice how your thoughts influence the intensity of the experience. Notice also how you behave in response to this exercise. Are you sitting back relaxed? Are you sitting forward in your chair, gripping the armrests? Are you fidgeting?

- Notice how different thoughts and different behaviors change the intensity of the bodily feelings you experience when doing these exercises.
- Do any of the exposures bring on bodily feelings similar to symptoms you sometimes feel? If so, you might benefit from engaging in the exposures repeatedly, as practice.

You can gradually lengthen the duration of your exposure to your bodily feelings so that the intensity of your feelings either remains the same or increases. You will notice, however, that the level of your distress eventually decreases as you become better able to endure the feelings. The same exposure exercise should be conducted repeatedly, with you only waiting long enough in between rounds of the exposure for the symptoms to mostly subside. You can then repeat this exercise until your distress reaches a 2 or less (on a scale of 0 to 8, as described above).

Worksheet 11.4: Bodily Feelings Exposure Practice, located near the end of this chapter, can be used to track your response to these exposures. After each exposure, rate the intensity of the bodily feelings you experience, distress associated with your bodily feelings, and similarity of those bodily feelings to those that typically occur as part of an emotional response. Rate each item on a scale from 0 to 8, with 0 = none, 4 = moderate, and 8 = extreme. Worksheet 11.4 is also available for download by searching for this book's title on the Oxford Academic platform at academic.oup.com.

Home Practice 2: Emotion Exposures to Approach Uncomfortable Situations

Box 11.1 can help you design and carry out an effective exposure. First, think back to the situations that you've been avoiding because of the unpleasant feelings they cause or that you worry they will cause. Choose one specific situation that you think you want to approach differently. Perhaps this is a situation that you've been avoiding. When approaching uncomfortable situations, it's important that the first situation you choose to approach isn't *too* uncomfortable—or *too easy*, for that matter. Ideally choose a situation that makes you feel just uncomfortable enough to feel reasonably challenged. Perhaps find a situation in the middle of your Emotion Exposure Ladder.

Any situation that you choose to approach should be a *safe* situation. You should not choose a situation in which you know that you could be physically harmed, attacked, assaulted, at risk of losing a basic need (e.g., housing, financial support), or otherwise harmed.

For other situations, such as having difficult conversations with friends or family, or meeting new potential dating partners, try approaching these situations using the same general steps you learned last chapter about being assertive:

1. Identify the challenging situation.
2. Challenge unassertive thoughts.
3. Act assertively.
4. Review what happened, whether you were able to be assertive regardless of the outcome, and the coping skills you used.

As you do the exposure exercise, you might find it helpful to write out your experience step by step on Worksheet 11.5: Record of Exposure Exercises, which is located at the end of this chapter and is also available for download by searching for this book's title on the Oxford Academic platform at academic.oup.com.

Key Things to Remember About Emotion Exposures

Practice, Practice, Practice!

It's especially important that you commit to making time and effort during this last part of treatment because this is where the greatest change may occur. You should try to set up several emotion exposures in a week. The more you can do, the better.

It may take a couple practices facing each situation before you begin to feel more comfortable. After all, you probably practiced avoiding that situation many times in the past—so it makes sense that it takes time to get used to facing these situations.

You Might Experience a Setback

Sometimes when you do an emotion exposure, you might find the emotions too difficult to experience and decide to stop the exposure early. Try not to get too discouraged—self-compassion is key here. You have had a lot of practice avoiding your emotions, and breaking that pattern takes time.

If you escape from the situation, give yourself a moment, and then get back in there. If you need to move a step down on the Emotion Exposure Ladder or change the emotion exposure to make it a little easier, go ahead.

It is also possible that the things you worry about during an emotion exposure will actually happen. You may have a panic attack, feel awkward in a social setting, or something else. Remember Dishon from the beginning of this chapter? Let's say Dishon tests out his theory by doing an emotion exposure and his worst fear comes true: He goes to a party, the gay men there ice him out, and he doesn't know how to connect with them. Instead of freezing up, Dishon can use the skills he learned from this treatment to prove to himself that he can handle it. He can show himself that his emotions don't have to control his behavior, and he has other options besides avoiding social events all together. Even if the men who were at the party weren't friendly, he still managed it. We don't consider that a bad thing. In fact, having times when an emotion exposure does not go as well as you wanted actually leads to more lasting progress in the long run.

Box 11.1. Guidelines for Designing and Carrying Out an Effective Exposure Exercise

1. Choose your task.
   - Pick a situation or an emotional experience that is going to *challenge* you, but don't try to do a task that is too difficult. Also, be sure to choose a situation that will not cause you harm.
   - The purpose of the exposure is to learn that you can master the situation or emotional experience, even in the face of very intense anxiety, fear, or depression.
   - Always complete exposure exercises without emotional behaviors (subtle or overt behavioral avoidance, cognitive avoidance, or safety signals), so make sure to do something that is manageable.
   - The higher the level of difficulty of the exposure exercises you can complete, the better you will feel in the long term.
2. Before the exposure exercise
   - Remind yourself that facing your emotions is the only way to make them more manageable.
   - Similarly, if you find that you "just don't want to do it" because you feel depressed or anxious, *this is the moment to push yourself even harder.* You cannot trust your emotions in this moment—remember that what goes up, must come down.

3. During the exposure exercise
   - Practice awareness of your thoughts, behaviors, and bodily feelings, and the situation around you.
   - Prevent yourself from engaging in any emotional behaviors (subtle or overt behavioral avoidance, cognitive avoidance, or safety signals). Don't try to push away uncomfortable thoughts and bodily feelings—they are there and must be experienced head on in order to change and to break the cycle.
   - Notice any emotional behaviors you might have the urge to engage in—and do not engage in them. You will be reinforcing the negative cycle of emotions if you do.
   - Stay in the situation until your emotional distress has reduced. Notice what it's like when your emotions are reducing on their own. See how you are able to make a choice about how you respond, instead of being driven by your feelings.
4. After the exposure exercise
   - Look back and evaluate how the situational exposure went.
   - Did what you fear would happen actually happen?
   - Did you do anything to prevent your emotions from becoming too intense (i.e., emotional behaviors)?
   - Did you stay in the emotion exposure long enough?
   - What could you have done to challenge yourself even more?
5. *If you find yourself avoiding the exposure exercise*, re-evaluate your fears by answering some of these questions:
   - What did you fear would happen?
   - What do you imagine happening that would be so terrible?
   - What would be so bad about that happening?
   - If you could be sure that it is all that would happen, would you still be as afraid of it as you are?

Make It Part of Your Routine

Since emotion exposures can sometimes be difficult to arrange and cause uncomfortable emotions, it can be easy to put them off. Scheduling a day and time for exposures is a helpful strategy. For example:

Angela avoided queer bars and spaces because she compared herself to the other women there and felt bad about herself. Being around that many queer people also reminded her of how uncomfortable she was with being bisexual.

When designing her emotion exposures, Angela scheduled times to go to a queer bar by herself for at least 30 minutes. At first, she started going at times when the bar wasn't busy. But over time, she scheduled her exposures for busier times like

Friday and Saturday nights. If she had not made a schedule ahead of time, Angela probably wouldn't have gone at all. She would not have had the chance to learn that she could handle it.

Avoid Avoidance

When doing emotion exposures, it's important to try to really feel the emotion and to "avoid avoiding." Think ahead about the most likely emotional behaviors you'll have the urge to engage in and plan what you will do instead.

The Attitude with Which You Approach the Task Can Be Important

Are you doing your emotion exposures reluctantly, just trying to get through them and wishing they were over? Or are you welcoming your own distress with courage and acceptance? Treat each emotion exposure as a chance to learn that your emotions are not as uncomfortable as you thought.

Overall Depression Severity and Interference Scale (ODSIS)

Instructions: The following items ask about depression. For each item, indicate the number for the answer that best describes your experience over the past week.

—1. In the past week, how often have you felt depressed?

0 = **No depression** in the past week.

1 = **Infrequent depression**. Felt depressed a few times.

2 = **Occasional depression**. Felt depressed as much of the time as not.

3 = **Frequent depression**. Felt depressed most of the time.

4 = **Constant depression**. Felt depressed all of the time.

—2. In the past week, when you have felt depressed, how intense or severe was your depression?

0 = **Little or None**: Depression was absent or barely noticeable.

1 = **Mild**: Depression was at a low level.

2 = **Moderate**: Depression was intense at times.

3 = **Severe**: Depression was intense much of the time.

4 = **Extreme**: Depression was overwhelming.

—3. In the past week, how often did you have difficulty engaging in or being interested in activities you normally enjoy because of depression?

0 = **None**: I had no difficulty engaging in or being interested in activities that I normally enjoy because of depression.

1 = **Infrequent**: A few times I had difficulty engaging in or being interested in activities that I normally enjoy because of depression. My lifestyle was not affected.

2 = **Occasional**: I had some difficulty engaging in or being interested in activities that I normally enjoy because of depression. My lifestyle has only changed in minor ways.

3 = **Frequent**: I have considerable difficulty engaging in or being interested in activities that I normally enjoy because of depression. I have made significant changes in my lifestyle because of being unable to become interested in activities I used to enjoy.

4 = **All the Time**: I have been unable to participate in or be interested in activities that I normally enjoy because of depression. My lifestyle has been extensively affected and I no longer do things that I used to enjoy.

—4. In the past week, how much did your depression interfere with your ability to do the things you needed to do at work, at school, or at home?

0 = **None**: No interference at work/home/school from depression.

1 = **Mild**: My depression has caused some interference at work/home/school. Things are more difficult, but everything that needs to be done is still getting done.

2 = **Moderate**: My depression definitely interferes with tasks. Most things are still getting done, but few things are being done as well as in the past.

3 = **Severe**: My depression has really changed my ability to get things done. Some tasks are still being done, but many things are not. My performance has definitely suffered.

4 = **Extreme**: My depression has become incapacitating. I am unable to complete tasks and have had to leave school, have quit or been fired from my job, or have been unable to complete tasks at home and have faced consequences like bill collectors, eviction, etc.

—5. In the past week, how much has depression interfered with your social life and relationships?

0 = **None**: My depression doesn't affect my relationships.

1 = **Mild**: My depression slightly interferes with my relationships. Some of my friendships and other relationships have suffered, but, overall, my social life is still fulfilling.

2 = **Moderate**: I have experienced some interference with my social life, but I still have a few close relationships. I don't spend as much time with others as in the past, but I still socialize sometimes.

3 = **Severe**: My friendships and other relationships have suffered a lot because of depression. I do not enjoy social activities. I socialize very little.

4 = **Extreme**: My depression has completely disrupted my social activities. All of my relationships have suffered or ended. My family life is extremely strained.

Total Score: ___

Overall Anxiety Severity and Interference Scale (OASIS)

Instructions: The following items ask about anxiety and fear. For each item, indicate the number for the answer that best describes your experience over the past week.

—1. In the past week, how often have you felt anxious?

    0 = **No anxiety** in the past week.

    1 = **Infrequent anxiety.** Felt anxious a few times.

    2 = **Occasional anxiety.** Felt anxious as much of the time as not. It was hard to relax.

    3 = **Frequent anxiety.** Felt anxious most of the time. It was very difficult to relax.

    4 = **Constant anxiety.** Felt anxious all of the time and never really relaxed.

—2. In the past week, when you have felt anxious, how intense or severe was your anxiety?

    0 = **Little or None:** Anxiety was absent or barely noticeable.

    1 = **Mild:** Anxiety was at a low level. It was possible to relax when I tried. Physical symptoms were only slightly uncomfortable.

    2 = **Moderate:** Anxiety was distressing at times. It was hard to relax or concentrate, but I could do it if I tried. Physical symptoms were uncomfortable.

    3 = **Severe:** Anxiety was intense much of the time. It was very difficult to relax or focus on anything else. Physical symptoms were extremely uncomfortable.

    4 = **Extreme:** Anxiety was overwhelming. It was impossible to relax at all. Physical symptoms were unbearable.

—3. In the past week, how often did you avoid situations, places, objects, or activities because of anxiety or fear?

    0 = **None:** I do not avoid places, situations, activities, or things because of fear.

    1 = **Infrequent:** I avoid something once in a while, but will usually face the situation or confront the object. My lifestyle is not affected.

    2 = **Occasional:** I have some fear of certain situations, places, or objects, but it is still manageable. My lifestyle has only changed in minor ways. I always or almost always avoid the things I fear when I'm alone, but can handle them if someone comes with me.

    3 = **Frequent:** I have considerable fear and really try to avoid the things that frighten me. I have made significant changes in my lifestyle to avoid the object, situation, activity, or place.

    4 = **All the Time:** Avoiding objects, situations, activities, or places has taken over my life. My lifestyle has been extensively affected and I no longer do things that I used to enjoy.

—4. In the past week, how much did your anxiety interfere with your ability to do the things you needed to do at work, at school, or at home?

    0 = **None:** No interference at work/home/school from anxiety.

    1 = **Mild:** My anxiety has caused some interference at work/home/school. Things are more difficult, but everything that needs to be done is still getting done.

2 = **Moderate:** My anxiety definitely interferes with tasks. Most things are still getting done, but few things are being done as well as in the past.

3 = **Severe:** My anxiety has really changed my ability to get things done. Some tasks are still being done, but many things are not. My performance has definitely suffered.

4 = **Extreme:** My anxiety has become incapacitating. I am unable to complete tasks and have had to leave school, have quit or been fired from my job, or have been unable to complete tasks at home and have faced consequences like bill collectors, eviction, etc.

—5. In the past week, how much has anxiety interfered with your social life and relationships?

0 = **None:** My anxiety doesn't affect my relationships.

1 = **Mild:** My anxiety slightly interferes with my relationships. Some of my friendships and other relationships have suffered, but, overall, my social life is still fulfilling.

2 = **Moderate:** I have experienced some interference with my social life, but I still have a few close relationships. I don't spend as much time with others as in the past, but I still socialize sometimes.

3 = **Severe:** My friendships and other relationships have suffered a lot because of anxiety. I do not enjoy social activities. I socialize very little.

4 = **Extreme:** My anxiety has completely disrupted my social activities. All of my relationships have suffered or ended. My family life is extremely strained.

Total Score: ___

Progress Record

ODSIS

```
20 ──────────────────────────────
18 ──────────────────────────────
16 ──────────────────────────────
14 ──────────────────────────────
12 ──────────────────────────────
10 ──────────────────────────────
 8 ──────────────────────────────
 6 ──────────────────────────────
 4 ──────────────────────────────
 2 ──────────────────────────────
 0 ──────────────────────────────
```

Week 1 2 3 4 5 6 7 8 9 10 11 12 13 14 15 16 17 18 19 20 21 22 23 24 v

OASIS

```
20 ──────────────────────────────
18 ──────────────────────────────
16 ──────────────────────────────
14 ──────────────────────────────
12 ──────────────────────────────
10 ──────────────────────────────
 8 ──────────────────────────────
 6 ──────────────────────────────
 4 ──────────────────────────────
 2 ──────────────────────────────
 0 ──────────────────────────────
```

Week 1 2 3 4 5 6 7 8 9 10 11 12 13 14 15 16 17 18 19 20 21 22 23 24 v

Other Assessment

```
20 ──────────────────────────────
18 ──────────────────────────────
16 ──────────────────────────────
14 ──────────────────────────────
12 ──────────────────────────────
10 ──────────────────────────────
 8 ──────────────────────────────
 6 ──────────────────────────────
 4 ──────────────────────────────
 2 ──────────────────────────────
 0 ──────────────────────────────
```

Week 1 2 3 4 5 6 7 8 9 10 11 12 13 14 15 16 17 18 19 20 21 22 23 24 v

Worksheet 11.1: Reviewing Your Progress

1. Have you been able to set time aside to practice mindfulness? Were you able to check in with yourself every morning and night? What obstacles have you noticed?

_____

_____

_____

2. Have you practiced identifying and challenging your automatic thoughts? Describe one situation where you used this technique.

_____

_____

_____

3. Have you continued to practice identifying emotion avoidance tendencies? Describe those tendencies.

_____

_____

_____

4. Describe a situation where you challenged an emotional behavior and what you did instead of avoiding emotions (for example, using emotional awareness/being mindful, facing the emotion, noticing automatic thoughts, and being flexible with your interpretations). What did you learn?

_____

_____

_____

Worksheet 11.2: Emotion Exposure Ladder

Do Not Avoid		Hesitate to Enter but Rarely Avoid		Sometimes Avoid		Usually Avoid		Always Avoid
0	1	2	3	4	5	6	7	8
No Distress		Slight Distress		Definite Distress		Strong Distress		Extreme Distress

Ranking	Description	Avoid	Distress
1. (Worst)			
2.			
3.			
4.			
5.			
6.			
7.			
8.			

	Do Not Avoid	Hesitate to Enter but Rarely Avoid		Sometimes Avoid		Usually Avoid		AlwaysAvoid
	1	2	3	4	5	6	7	8
	No Distress	Slight Distress		Definite Distress		Strong Distress		Extreme Distress

Ranking	Description	Avoid	Distress
1. (Worst)	Asking a guy out in person	8	8
2.	Getting a guy's number	7	8
3.	Talking to queer guys in public spaces	7	7
4.	Flirting with queer guys in public spaces	7	6
5.	Going on a date	5	6
6.	Setting up a date	5	4
7.	Messaging guys online	4	4
8.	Creating an online dating profile	4	3

Figure 11.1

Miguel's Completed Emotion Exposure Ladder

Worksheet 11.3: Bodily Feelings Exposure Test (For People Who Fear Bodily Feelings)

Please complete each of the exposures (as described in this chapter) below. Be sure to engage in each exposure fully and try to produce at least moderate intensity of the bodily feelings. After the exposure, be sure to note:

1. The **bodily feelings** you experienced
2. The **intensity** of the bodily feelings (0–8 scale; 0 = no intensity, 8 = extreme intensity)
3. The level of **distress** you experienced during the exposure (0–8 scale; 0 = no distress, 8 = extreme distress)
4. The degree of **similarity to your naturally occurring bodily feelings** (0–8 scale; 0 = not at all similar, 8 = extremely similar)

Wait until the bodily feelings have mostly subsided before attempting the next exposure. Use the other spaces provided to be creative and come up with additional exposures that are specific to you. When you are done, pick three of the exposures that produced the most anxiety for you. Put a star next to those.

Procedure	Bodily Feelings Experienced	Intensity	Distress	Similarity
Breathing through thin straw (2 minutes)				
Spinning while standing or in a swivel chair (60 seconds)				
Running in place (60 seconds)				
Other: (___ seconds)				
Other: (___ seconds)				

Worksheet 11.4: Bodily Feelings Exposure Practice (For People Who Fear Bodily Feelings)

DAY 1: _____

Trial	Intensity	Distress	Similarity
1.			
2.			
3.			
4.			
5.			

DAY 2: _____

Trial	Intensity	Distress	Similarity
1.			
2.			
3.			
4.			
5.			

DAY 3: _____

Trial	Intensity	Distress	Similarity
1.			
2.			
3.			
4.			
5.			

DAY 4: _____

Trial	Intensity	Distress	Similarity
1.			
2.			
3.			
4.			
5.			

DAY 5: _____

Trial	Intensity	Distress	Similarity
1.			
2.			
3.			
4.			
5.			

DAY 6: _____

Trial	Intensity	Distress	Similarity
1.			
2.			
3.			
4.			
5.			

Worksheet 11.5: Record of Exposure Exercises

Exposure Situation or Emotion:

_____

Prior to the exposure:

Anticipatory Distress (0–8): _____

Thoughts, Behaviors, and Bodily Feelings you noticed before the exposure:

_____

_____

_____

Re-evaluate your automatic thoughts about the exposure:

_____

_____

_____

After completing the exposure:

Thoughts, Behaviors, and Bodily Feelings you noticed during the exposure:

_____

_____

_____

Number of minutes you did the exposure: _____

Maximum distress during the exposure (0–8): _____

Distress at the end of the exposure (0–8): _____

Any attempts to avoid your emotions (i.e., emotional behaviors—behavioral avoidance, cognitive avoidance, or safety signals)?

_____

_____

_____

What did you take away from this exposure exercise? Did your feared outcomes occur? If so, how were you able to cope with them?

_____

_____

_____

CHAPTER 12

Module 9: Recognizing Accomplishments and Looking to the Future

Chapter 12 Overview

You made it to the end of this treatment program—congratulations! The main goal for today is for you to see how you now have tools to cope with LGBTQ-related stress and other difficulties on your own. You'll also think about what your goals are for the future and how you can use the skills you've learned in this treatment program to help you get there. You've got this!

Chapter 12 Outline

- Weekly Check-In
- Review Home Practice from Chapter 11
- Review Your Progress
- Plan for Future Challenges
- Review Your New Skills
- Plan for Continued Practice
- Set Long-Term Goals
- Share Your Resilience
- Looking Back and Looking Forward
- Summary
- Continued Home Practice

Take a minute to track your symptoms using the ODSIS and OASIS, located at the end of this chapter. You may also photocopy these forms or download multiple copies by searching for this book's title on the Oxford Academic platform at academic.oup.com. Do you notice any changes? What do you attribute these changes to?

Review Home Practice from Chapter 11

Before beginning this last chapter, take a look at Worksheet 11.5: Record of Exposure Exercises from the last chapter. If you also practiced exposing yourself to uncomfortable bodily feelings, go ahead and take a look at completed Worksheet 11.3: Bodily Feelings Exposure Test and Worksheet 11.4: Bodily Feelings Exposure Practice as well.

First, acknowledge the hard work it took to do these exposures. Exposures are meant to be challenging, and you probably had to deal with some discomfort to try them out. Even if your exposures didn't go as planned, take a moment to recognize that you challenged yourself by taking on these exposures.

Now, let's reflect on how these exposures went for you:

- What uncomfortable feelings or challenging situations did you intentionally seek out?
- How did your emotions change through the exposure? What did you notice about your emotions during the situation?
- What did you learn about these situations or about your reactions from doing these exposures?
- Did you engage in any emotional behaviors during the exposures?
- Were you able to stay present and nonjudgmental (i.e., mindfully aware) during the exposures?
- What challenges did you face while doing these exposures?

Sometimes, doing an emotion exposure or an internal exposure doesn't work out as planned. For example, maybe your emotional experience did not change during the emotion exposure. There are a couple of reasons why this could happen:

1. *Engaging in emotional behaviors during the exposure:* Emotional behaviors (e.g., avoidance strategies) can be so practiced and subtle that it can be hard to do an emotion exposure without engaging in them. You might also engage in your emotional behaviors without even realizing that you are doing them. Next time you try an exposure, try checking in for any emotional behaviors you may be engaging in, as these can detract from the impact of the exposure.

2. *Choosing an exposure that is too high or too low on your emotion exposure ladder:* If you chose something too high on your ladder (something that is too anxiety provoking), you can simply try an exposure next time that is lower, which is likely to be more successful. By slowly working your way up to that higher exposure, you can build on your past successes (see Box 12.1 for an example of this). In contrast, sometimes to prevent feeling overwhelmed, people will choose an exposure that is too low—that is, not challenging enough—on their ladder. This is not helpful either, as it prevents you from experiencing the strong emotions that the exposure is meant to elicit. If you chose an exposure too low on the ladder, next time you can try an exposure that is higher on the ladder.

Box 12.1. Adjusting an Emotion Exposure Within the Ladder

Andrew, who is also completing this treatment program, decided to do an emotion exposure of asking Matt out on a date. While getting ready for the exposure, Andrew noticed that the idea of seeing Matt made him anxious and insecure to the point of feeling as though he had nothing to offer. Andrew took a step back from his first exposure and came up with a different, more achievable exposure: He decided to say hello to Matt the next time he saw him, and to start a conversation. Adjusting his experiment made Andrew feel more confident. It also helped him get to know Matt a little bit more. In the end, it was actually Matt who asked Andrew out on a date!

As you approach the end of this treatment, you may be feeling excited because you've seen improvements in your symptoms. You may also feel disappointed if you haven't seen as much improvement as you had hoped.

It is important to remember that the goal of this program is to teach you helpful skills for responding to your emotions, including those that are triggered or made worse by LGBTQ-related stress situations. Although it is very common for people to have made some noticeable progress, this treatment program is short, and there is still room to improve after treatment ends. In fact, for most people, continued progress is expected. This is because it takes time after learning these skills to see the full effect. Remember that this program was designed not only for progress right now, but to teach you skills to continue using in the future as well.

Compared to when you started this program, what have you gained? What changes have you made? The following questions may help you reflect on the progress you've made:

- How were you feeling when you started? Where are you now?
- What kinds of not-so-helpful coping were you doing when you started? Where are you now?
- Look at your Progress Record, where you have been tracking your weekly responses to the ODSIS and OASIS. What do you notice in terms of patterns throughout this treatment program?
- Try completing Worksheet 12.1: Assessing Changes During the Treatment Program to further explore how things may have changed from the beginning of this treatment program to now. The worksheet is located at the end of this chapter and is also available for download by searching for this book's title on the Oxford Academic platform at academic.oup.com.

It's important to acknowledge the changes you have accomplished, no matter how big or small. You can hopefully now see that you can cope with challenges better than you initially thought.

Change takes time and practice, and can be difficult, as well as highly rewarding. Most importantly, it takes patience and nonjudgmental awareness.

In case you're not feeling like you're making progress, try going back to previous chapters to refresh and practice your skills. As you go back to

Table 12.1. Common Barriers to Treatment Progress and Potential Solutions

Barriers to Treatment Progress	Potential Solutions
☒ Setting goals that are abstract, unrealistic, or long term	☑ Go back to the earlier sessions and Worksheet 4.3: Treatment Goal Setting Worksheet, and scale back your goals so they are more (1) concrete, (2) realistic given the time frame and situation you are in, and (3) achievable in the short term.
☒ Not having enough time to practice the skills (i.e., reading the workbook but not trying out the home practice exercises)	☑ Set aside a weekly practice time so that you can try out the home practice exercises. Home practice exercises are not always time-consuming, and you can usually integrate them into your normal daily activities. Consider brainstorming ideas for practicing with trusted family or friends (or a therapist, if you are working with one).
☒ Not feeling motivated to engage with the treatment program or the home practice exercises, or feeling overwhelmed by them	☑ As discussed at the beginning of the treatment program, it's normal for motivation to go up and down throughout treatment. This can be especially true when you feel depressed, anxious, or too tired since these feelings can get in the way of practicing. Try going back to Worksheet 4.1: Decisional Balance Worksheet to identify your reasons for changing, or try revisiting your treatment goals on Worksheet 4.3: Treatment Goal Setting Worksheet, to decide what you want to get out of treatment. The exercises contained in both of these worksheets can be very helpful for boosting motivation, especially when the home practice exercises get more challenging. Sharing with a trusted family member, friend, or therapist can also help to boost motivation.
☒ Not fully understanding the treatment program, exercises, or treatment principles	☑ Remember that this is all new! It's normal for learning new material to take some time. If you're working with a therapist, try sharing that you're feeling confused. If you're completing the workbook on your own, try going back and revisiting earlier chapters (they may make more sense the second time through) or, if you have a friend you trust, you can go through the workbook with them and discuss together the areas that are more confusing.

these earlier chapters, think about whether any of the common barriers and potential solutions listed in Table 12.1 may be relevant to you.

Remember: Lack of progress is not hopeless. Once you explore the reasons that may have gotten in the way of progress, you can problem solve!

Plan for Future Challenges

Everyone has ups and downs in their emotional life. It is certain that you will have intense, uncomfortable emotions in the future, in response either to LGBTQ-related stress or to other life stressors. In the same way that you are more likely to get sick when you are under a lot of stress, you are more likely to fall back into old patterns of avoiding your emotions when under a lot of stress. Sometimes, however, it may seem like your mental health symptoms flare up when there hasn't been an increase in stress. Even though this can be very upsetting, these ups and downs are normal and do not necessarily mean that you have fallen back into old patterns and lost the skills you had gained or that your ways of experiencing your emotions will be just as difficult as they were before you started this treatment.

The skills that you learned to manage your emotions in this treatment also apply to coping with these ups and downs in the future. For instance, responding to an increase in symptoms with self-criticism and self-judgment will only make the symptoms worse. It is very easy to jump to conclusions and think the worst when symptoms flare up. You may find yourself thinking that treatment failed or that you'll never be able to cope with these intense emotions.

Thinking about the treatment skills we've covered in this program:

- What specific triggers do you think might cause distress or a sense of "relapse"?

_____

_____

- What is your plan for managing that distress?

_____

_____

- What strategies can you use to cope? Think about the skills you've learned in this treatment program. What seemed to work?

_____

_____

Continuing to practice the treatment skills—regardless of whether your symptoms flare up again—is important, as this continued practice will solidify the learning and gains that you made in treatment. Similarly, if you find that your symptoms are increasing again, it can be helpful to revisit the skills from this treatment program and begin practicing them more intentionally, as you did when actively engaging in the treatment program.

Review Your New Skills

We have shared a lot of information over the course of this treatment program about how to be more accepting of your emotions. You were introduced to techniques and skills that you can use to respond to uncomfortable emotions that happen in the future, including:

- Mindfulness and nonjudgmental awareness,
- Changing your automatic thoughts,
- Communicating assertively, and
- Situational exposures and bodily feelings exposures.

Each of these skills has been shown to help people who experience depression, anxiety, and other difficult emotions. Now you have a whole new coping kit to help you approach situations that may have been really hard to navigate in the past!

As you transition to the end of this workbook, it can be helpful to reflect on the treatment skills you have learned, and how you might apply them to future challenges. Consider:

- What skills have you found most helpful?

_____

_____

- What skills come most easily to you?

_____

_____

- What skills do you feel like you could use more practice with?

_____

_____

- Think about a future situation that might be challenging for you. How could you apply the skills you've learned in treatment to that situation?

_____

_____

Here are some of the most important takeaway messages from this workbook:

- All emotions, even the ones that feel negative or uncomfortable, give you important information that can motivate you to act in helpful ways.
- Staying present in the moment and being nonjudgmental of your emotions can help stop emotions from getting super-intense.
- The way you think about a situation changes how you feel, and how you feel affects the way you interpret a situation.
- Although avoiding uncomfortable emotions can work well in the short term, it isn't an effective long-term coping strategy (and can even make things worse).

To help you remember all of your new skills, we created an action plan for you to use whenever you notice a negative emotion starting to build. This plan, shown in Box 12.2, is based on the three-component model of emotions, introduced in Chapter 6 of this treatment program, to help you remember it.

Plan for Continued Practice

Even though you are finishing this treatment program, promoting your well-being and progress is an ongoing process. The single most effective way to maintain the progress you have made so far and to keep improving is to continue to practice the skills you've learned. Keep in mind that even if you have made a lot of progress so far, these are newly learned behaviors that will require time and effort in order to "stick."

If you look at Worksheet 12.2: Practice Plan, you'll notice several possible areas for change, such as present-focused emotional awareness, increasing flexible thinking, reducing avoidance and changing emotional behaviors,

> **Box 12.2. Skills Action Plan**
>
> Do a quick three-point check. Use your breath or other cue as an anchor to help bring you out of your head and to anchor yourself in the present moment.
>
> **1. What are you _thinking right now?_** What negative automatic thoughts are you having right now? Are you jumping to conclusions or thinking the worst? Are you responding to a past concern or future worry? Are there any other ways to interpret this situation that may be more helpful? What are some skills you can use to cope?
>
> **2. What are you _feeling in your body right now?_** What physical feelings are you noticing? Are you tired, hungry, or rundown? Are your physical feelings making your emotions more intense, or the other way around? Try to stay in the present moment with your physical feelings without trying to control them or to distract yourself.
>
> **3. What are you _doing now, or what do you feel like doing right now?_** Are you avoiding a situation that may cause an uncomfortable emotion? Remember that challenging an emotion-driven behavior involves causing uncomfortable emotions and doing helpful _alternate actions._

as well as emotion exposures. Studies have shown that people are more likely to take action when they plan it out in advance. The worksheet is located at the end of this chapter and is also available for download by searching for this book's title on the Oxford Academic platform at academic.oup.com.

Worksheet 12.2: Practice Plan asks you to come up with a plan for how you can practice each skill. Even with the best of intentions, it is hard to follow through with a practice plan unless you get specific about exactly how and when you will practice.

Take Elana, for example:

Elana planned to work on approaching, instead of avoiding, emotions by not using distraction as a coping strategy during their commute to work, when they usually feel anxious/depressed. However, since this plan does not specify when or how they will stop using distraction, Elana had a very hard time keeping up with this plan. That is, until they reworked their plan: _"When I take the subway to and from work, I won't listen to music or read on my phone to distract myself. At each subway stop, I will take a deep breath to anchor myself in the present moment."_

What do *you* want to practice and work on in the coming weeks, after treatment ends? Try to be as clear as you can in your descriptions, just like Elana. Setting aside time each week to review your progress and continuing to set smaller goals can help you achieve your long-term goals. What seemed to help you during the treatment program? Present-focused emotion awareness, or perhaps reducing avoidance and changing emotional behaviors? What new techniques have you been using? What changes can you create to make your future better? An example practice plan is shown in Table 12.2, which can be found near the end of this chapter.

Now that you have a new set of skills and are more aware of your emotions, you can notice when your symptoms get worse and do something effective to manage them. This can be especially helpful right after treatment, but you can continue the practice plan for as long as you find it helpful.

You now have the tools to be your own therapist!

Set Long-Term Goals

With treatment ending, another strategy for promoting your ongoing growth and use of these treatment skills is to think about and set some long-term goals. You've worked hard to get into the practice of making positive changes in your life over the past few months, so now is a great time to keep building on this practice.

Similar to Worksheet 4.3: Treatment Goal Setting Worksheet, which you completed early in this treatment program, you can now start working towards new long-term goals.

Why Set Long-Term Goals? Where Do You Start?

Setting goals is a critical part of making changes to your life and staying motivated.

- Take a look at the treatment goals you've completed since the beginning of this program. Now that you have completed this treatment, you may have made lots of progress on some of the goals you set.

- To stay motivated, take a moment to revisit your goals and update them if necessary. You can use Worksheet 12.3: Long-Term Goals to record these updated goals as you also start thinking about new future goals for yourself. The worksheet is located at the end of this chapter and is also available for download by searching for this book's title on the Oxford Academic platform at academic.oup.com.

Now that you might be feeling better and more prepared, additional possibilities may seem open to you (like starting to date, going back to school, or looking for a new job). Using Worksheet 12.3: Long-Term Goals, think about things you would like to achieve, and the steps you would need to take to achieve these goals. As you are updating your goals on this worksheet, remember that people tend to feel most motivated when working towards something that is important to them. What is personally meaningful to you? Once you have some updated goals in mind, ask yourself the following questions:

- Are your goals specific and concrete enough for you to easily measure your progress?
- Are your goals manageable and realistic? Remember that the purpose of goals is to motivate you. If you set goals that are unrealistic, you will most likely end up feeling defeated.
- Is the ability to achieve your goals within your control, or is it possible that you would fail for reasons beyond your control? For instance, if you set a goal to go on two dates next month, achieving the goal may be out of your control. However, if you revise your goal to talking to someone new on a dating app each week, you can control whether you achieve that goal.

Share Your Resilience

You are resilient! And it can help to see your resilience in action. The last thing for you to do as part of this program is to use the skills you've learned to imagine helping someone else. Here are some stories where someone else is dealing with LGBTQ-related stress. Choose one that speaks to you, and take some time, using Worksheet 12.4: Sharing Your Resilience, to write to this person, telling them about your own experiences with LGBTQ-related stress, how you've handled it, and what coping strategies you find most helpful. By giving advice to another person in the letter you write, you might be reminded that you yourself are resilient and belong to a larger community of LGBTQ people. The worksheet is located at the end of this chapter and is also available for download by searching for this book's title on the Oxford Academic platform at academic.oup.com.

Alex

Alex is a non-binary student at a local high school. Alex recently came out to their dad, who responded by saying, "You're not gonna be non-binary under my roof!" He kicked them out and they have been couch-surfing since. That was several months ago, and they're still feeling really hopeless. They knew he wouldn't take the news well, but Alex never expected him to freak out this badly. Now Alex is worried about being homeless forever and how they will pay for college. And they're terrified that their dad will never speak to them again.

Imagine Alex comes to you for help. Based on your experiences, what advice would you give Alex on how to handle this situation? Write a message to them for 20 minutes about what you might say. Just follow your train of thought wherever it goes, without worrying about spelling, grammar, or structure. Please write for the whole 20 minutes. After you are done writing, read it over and reflect on the helpful, skillful advice you provided Alex.

Micah

Micah is a devout bisexual Christian man in his mid-20s. He has belonged to his church for his whole life and loves playing in the church band each Sunday. However, things have changed since he came out. His band members told him he's going to hell and kicked him out. His pastor asked him to meet so they could "pray it away." And everyone else at church gives him dirty looks like he's an abomination. So, he's stopped going. But now there's a big hole in Micah's life where his church life used to be, and he's worried that he'll never find a church community again.

Imagine Micah comes to you for help. Based on your experiences, what advice would you give him on how to handle this situation? Write a message to him for 20 minutes about what you might say. Just follow your train of thought wherever it goes, without worrying about spelling, grammar, or structure. Please write for the whole 20 minutes. After you are done writing, read it over and reflect on the helpful, skillful advice you provided Micah.

Natalie

Natalie is a high school student. A few months back, some students found out that she is lesbian, and she has been bullied and teased ever since, and her friends constantly tell jokes about gay people. Although several teachers see what's going on, they never intervene, and none are openly LGBTQ. She can't transfer schools and is feeling hopeless about ever being accepted for who she is.

Imagine Natalie comes to you for help. Based on your experiences, what advice would you give her on how to handle this situation? Write a message to her for 20 minutes about what you might say. Just follow your train of thought wherever it goes, without worrying about spelling, grammar, or structure. Please write for the whole 20 minutes. After you are done writing, read it over and reflect on the helpful, skillful advice you provided Natalie.

After you've finished writing, be sure to take a minute to reflect on what you think about what you wrote in your letter. What new strengths and resilience do you see in yourself now compared to when you started treatment? How can you use this new competence you've shown going forward in your life?

Looking Back and Looking Forward

We'd like to leave you with a few reminders as you continue to develop these skills and carry them with you through your own development as an LGBTQ person.

First, it takes both time and effort to change your response to stressful experiences and uncomfortable emotions, including those resulting from LGBTQ-related stress. Just as unhelpful ways of coping with intense emotions aren't learned overnight, it is unrealistic to expect that these unhelpful coping strategies will completely disappear right away. However, over time, consistent practice will allow you to replace unhelpful coping strategies with more helpful ones and change the way you respond to your emotions so that you can feel safe, strong, and confident.

Second, life will have its ups and downs, as it always does. The goal of this treatment has not been to eliminate the downs and amplify the ups. Instead, by practicing and strengthening your *approaches* to these ups and downs, we hope that you can be better able to enjoy the ups as they come, and better able to make it through the downs when they inevitably come too. You might even find that your high moments are a little bit higher, and your low moments are a little less low.

Finally, we want to remind you of something we shared early in this journey: Resilience and growth are often forged in the fires of adversity, which is why LGBTQ people possess unique strengths. The fact that you read this workbook means that you also have overcome major challenges in your life and are resilient. You can continue to draw upon this strength and resilience to keep bringing the skills from this program into your everyday life. We wish you the best of luck in your continued journey.

Summary

In this chapter you reviewed all the different skills you learned in this workbook and reflected on all the gains that you made during this treatment program. You also considered how you can continue to incorporate and practice the skills you learned in future challenges and to help you reach your long-term goals. Congratulations, you've completed this treatment program!

Continued Home Practice

You have reached the end of the workbook, but you can continue to practice the skills from this program. Here are some ideas for continuing your home practice:

- Practice nonjudgmental awareness and mindfulness every day.
- Continue identifying and challenging your automatic thoughts.
- Recognize and challenge emotion avoidance strategies.
- Practice identifying and challenging emotional behaviors.
- Practice communicating assertively.
- Continue to face challenging situations.
- Practice inducing bodily feelings.
- Fill in Worksheet 12.2: Practice Plan and Worksheet 12.3: Long-Term Goals.

Overall Depression Severity and Interference Scale (ODSIS)

Instructions: The following items ask about depression. For each item, indicate the number for the answer that best describes your experience over the past week.

—1. In the past week, how often have you felt depressed?

    0 = **No depression** in the past week.

    1 = **Infrequent depression**. Felt depressed a few times.

    2 = **Occasional depression**. Felt depressed as much of the time as not.

    3 = **Frequent depression**. Felt depressed most of the time.

    4 = **Constant depression**. Felt depressed all of the time.

—2. In the past week, when you have felt depressed, how intense or severe was your depression?

    0 = **Little or None**: Depression was absent or barely noticeable.

    1 = **Mild**: Depression was at a low level.

    2 = **Moderate**: Depression was intense at times.

    3 = **Severe**: Depression was intense much of the time.

    4 = **Extreme**: Depression was overwhelming.

—3. In the past week, how often did you have difficulty engaging in or being interested in activities you normally enjoy because of depression?

    0 = **None**: I had no difficulty engaging in or being interested in activities that I normally enjoy because of depression.

    1 = **Infrequent**: A few times I had difficulty engaging in or being interested in activities that I normally enjoy because of depression. My lifestyle was not affected.

    2 = **Occasional**: I had some difficulty engaging in or being interested in activities that I normally enjoy because of depression. My lifestyle has only changed in minor ways.

    3 = **Frequent**: I have considerable difficulty engaging in or being interested in activities that I normally enjoy because of depression. I have made significant changes in my lifestyle because of being unable to become interested in activities I used to enjoy.

    4 = **All the Time**: I have been unable to participate in or be interested in activities that I normally enjoy because of depression. My lifestyle has been extensively affected and I no longer do things that I used to enjoy.

—4. In the past week, how much did your depression interfere with your ability to do the things you needed to do at work, at school, or at home?

    0 = **None**: No interference at work/home/school from depression.

    1 = **Mild**: My depression has caused some interference at work/home/school. Things are more difficult, but everything that needs to be done is still getting done.

    2 = **Moderate**: My depression definitely interferes with tasks. Most things are still getting done, but few things are being done as well as in the past.

    3 = **Severe**: My depression has really changed my ability to get things done. Some tasks are still being done, but many things are not. My performance has definitely suffered.

4 = **Extreme**: My depression has become incapacitating. I am unable to complete tasks and have had to leave school, have quit or been fired from my job, or have been unable to complete tasks at home and have faced consequences like bill collectors, eviction, etc.

—5. In the past week, how much has depression interfered with your social life and relationships?

0 = **None**: My depression doesn't affect my relationships.

1 = **Mild**: My depression slightly interferes with my relationships. Some of my friendships and other relationships have suffered, but, overall, my social life is still fulfilling.

2 = **Moderate**: I have experienced some interference with my social life, but I still have a few close relationships. I don't spend as much time with others as in the past, but I still socialize sometimes.

3 = **Severe**: My friendships and other relationships have suffered a lot because of depression. I do not enjoy social activities. I socialize very little.

4 = **Extreme**: My depression has completely disrupted my social activities. All of my relationships have suffered or ended. My family life is extremely strained.

Total Score: ____

Overall Anxiety Severity and Interference Scale (OASIS)

Instructions: The following items ask about anxiety and fear. For each item, indicate the number for the answer that best describes your experience over the past week.

—1. In the past week, how often have you felt anxious?

0 = **No anxiety** in the past week.

1 = **Infrequent anxiety.** Felt anxious a few times.

2 = **Occasional anxiety.** Felt anxious as much of the time as not. It was hard to relax.

3 = **Frequent anxiety.** Felt anxious most of the time. It was very difficult to relax.

4 = **Constant anxiety.** Felt anxious all of the time and never really relaxed.

—2. In the past week, when you have felt anxious, how intense or severe was your anxiety?

0 = **Little or None:** Anxiety was absent or barely noticeable.

1 = **Mild:** Anxiety was at a low level. It was possible to relax when I tried. Physical symptoms were only slightly uncomfortable.

2 = **Moderate:** Anxiety was distressing at times. It was hard to relax or concentrate, but I could do it if I tried. Physical symptoms were uncomfortable.

3 = **Severe:** Anxiety was intense much of the time. It was very difficult to relax or focus on anything else. Physical symptoms were extremely uncomfortable.

4 = **Extreme:** Anxiety was overwhelming. It was impossible to relax at all. Physical symptoms were unbearable.

—3. In the past week, how often did you avoid situations, places, objects, or activities because of anxiety or fear?

0 = **None:** I do not avoid places, situations, activities, or things because of fear.

1 = **Infrequent:** I avoid something once in a while, but will usually face the situation or confront the object. My lifestyle is not affected.

2 = **Occasional:** I have some fear of certain situations, places, or objects, but it is still manageable. My lifestyle has only changed in minor ways. I always or almost always avoid the things I fear when I'm alone, but can handle them if someone comes with me.

3 = **Frequent:** I have considerable fear and really try to avoid the things that frighten me. I have made significant changes in my lifestyle to avoid the object, situation, activity, or place.

4 = **All the Time:** Avoiding objects, situations, activities, or places has taken over my life. My lifestyle has been extensively affected and I no longer do things that I used to enjoy.

—4. In the past week, how much did your anxiety interfere with your ability to do the things you needed to do at work, at school, or at home?

0 = **None:** No interference at work/home/school from anxiety.

1 = **Mild:** My anxiety has caused some interference at work/home/school. Things are more difficult, but everything that needs to be done is still getting done.

2 = **Moderate:** My anxiety definitely interferes with tasks. Most things are still getting done, but few things are being done as well as in the past.

3 = **Severe:** My anxiety has really changed my ability to get things done. Some tasks are still being done, but many things are not. My performance has definitely suffered.

4 = **Extreme:** My anxiety has become incapacitating. I am unable to complete tasks and have had to leave school, have quit or been fired from my job, or have been unable to complete tasks at home and have faced consequences like bill collectors, eviction, etc.

—5. In the past week, how much has anxiety interfered with your social life and relationships?

0 = **None:** My anxiety doesn't affect my relationships.

1 = **Mild:** My anxiety slightly interferes with my relationships. Some of my friendships and other relationships have suffered, but, overall, my social life is still fulfilling.

2 = **Moderate:** I have experienced some interference with my social life, but I still have a few close relationships. I don't spend as much time with others as in the past, but I still socialize sometimes.

3 = **Severe:** My friendships and other relationships have suffered a lot because of anxiety. I do not enjoy social activities. I socialize very little.

4 = **Extreme:** My anxiety has completely disrupted my social activities. All of my relationships have suffered or ended. My family life is extremely strained.

Total Score: ___

Progress Record

ODSIS

```
20 ─────────────────────────────────────────────
18 ─────────────────────────────────────────────
16 ─────────────────────────────────────────────
14 ─────────────────────────────────────────────
12 ─────────────────────────────────────────────
10 ─────────────────────────────────────────────
 8 ─────────────────────────────────────────────
 6 ─────────────────────────────────────────────
 4 ─────────────────────────────────────────────
 2 ─────────────────────────────────────────────
 0 ─────────────────────────────────────────────
```

Week 1 2 3 4 5 6 7 8 9 10 11 12 13 14 15 16 17 18 19 20 21 22 23 24 v

OASIS

```
20 ─────────────────────────────────────────────
18 ─────────────────────────────────────────────
16 ─────────────────────────────────────────────
14 ─────────────────────────────────────────────
12 ─────────────────────────────────────────────
10 ─────────────────────────────────────────────
 8 ─────────────────────────────────────────────
 6 ─────────────────────────────────────────────
 4 ─────────────────────────────────────────────
 2 ─────────────────────────────────────────────
 0 ─────────────────────────────────────────────
```

Week 1 2 3 4 5 6 7 8 9 10 11 12 13 14 15 16 17 18 19 20 21 22 23 24 v

Other Assessment

```
20 ─────────────────────────────────────────────
18 ─────────────────────────────────────────────
16 ─────────────────────────────────────────────
14 ─────────────────────────────────────────────
12 ─────────────────────────────────────────────
10 ─────────────────────────────────────────────
 8 ─────────────────────────────────────────────
 6 ─────────────────────────────────────────────
 4 ─────────────────────────────────────────────
 2 ─────────────────────────────────────────────
 0 ─────────────────────────────────────────────
```

Week 1 2 3 4 5 6 7 8 9 10 11 12 13 14 15 16 17 18 19 20 21 22 23 24 v

Worksheet 12.1: Assessing Changes During the Treatment Program

How have things changed with your overall feelings and life in general (e.g., general anxiety, social anxiety, depression, relationships with family/friends/colleagues/romantic partners)?	
Then:	
Now:	
How have things changed with the coping skills you use (e.g., avoiding social events, not talking to parents, risky sex, isolation, heavy drinking/drug use)?	
Then:	
Now:	
What do you want to continue working on?	

Worksheet 12.2: Practice Plan

Things to Practice	Description (How I Will Practice)
Present-Focused Emotion Awareness	
Increasing Cognitive Flexibility	
Reducing and Changing Emotional Behaviors	
Assertiveness	
Emotion Exposures	

Table 12.2. Example Practice Plan

Things to Practice	Description (How I Will Practice)
Present-Focused Emotion Awareness	If I start feeling anxious when I get ready for a date, I'll try to just let myself feel it and not judge myself for feeling that way.
Increasing Cognitive Flexibility	The next time I start procrastinating because I feel like I need to do something perfect, I can identify the "unhelpful thought" I'm having and try to come up with a more helpful thought.
Reducing and Changing Emotional Behaviors	Try going out to an LGBTQ event and only drinking soda to see what it's like to be in that kind of space without drinking alcohol, my go-to emotional behavior.
Assertiveness	Having an honest conversation with my friend about how it makes me feel when she jokes about my sexual identity.
Emotion Exposures	I'm ready to go to the next experiment on my Emotion Exposure Ladder: breathing through a straw until I feel like I'm hyperventilating and allowing myself to feel those bodily feelings without judgment.

Worksheet 12.3: Long-Term Goals

Long-Term Goals	Steps to Achieve Long-Term Goals

Worksheet 12.4: Sharing Your Resilience

Dear_____,

_____

_____

_____

_____

_____

_____

_____

_____

_____

_____

_____

_____

_____

_____

_____

John E. Pachankis, **PhD**, is the Susan Dwight Bliss Professor of Public Health and Psychiatry at Yale and Director of Yale's LGBTQ Mental Health Initiative. His research examines the mental health of LGBTQ populations globally and the efficacy of LGBTQ-affirmative mental health interventions. He has published 150+ scientific papers on LGBTQ mental health and stigma and recently co-edited the *Handbook of Evidence-Based Mental Health Practice with Sexual and Gender Minorities*, published by Oxford University Press.

Skyler D. Jackson, **PhD**, is an Associate Research Scientist at Yale School of Public Health. As an award-winning researcher and psychologist, his work examines how experiences of stigma—if not adequately coped with—interfere with psychological functioning and contribute to health disparities. In particular, much of his published work helps illuminate the complex role of intersectional stigma in shaping the everyday lives and health outcomes of LGBTQ people of color.

Audrey R. Harkness, **PhD**, is Assistant Professor of Public Health Sciences at the University of Miami. Her research focuses on mental health of LGBTQ populations, including mental health in the context of HIV prevention and treatment, mental health disparities and equity, and Latino/a/x LGBTQ communities in particular.

Steven A. Safren, **PhD**, is a Professor of Psychology and Cooper Fellow at the University of Miami (UM) in the Department of Psychology. He is also Director of the UM Center for HIV and Research in Mental Health (CHARM). For over 20 years, Dr. Safren has studied behavioral health related to sexual and gender minorities, much of which in the context of HIV prevention and treatment, both domestically and globally. He is a leading expert in cognitive behavioral therapy, has been the editor of the journal *Cognitive and Behavioral Practice*, and has published over 400 peer-reviewed papers in his field.